495/-

Kama Sutra
Feminine Pleasures
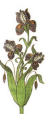

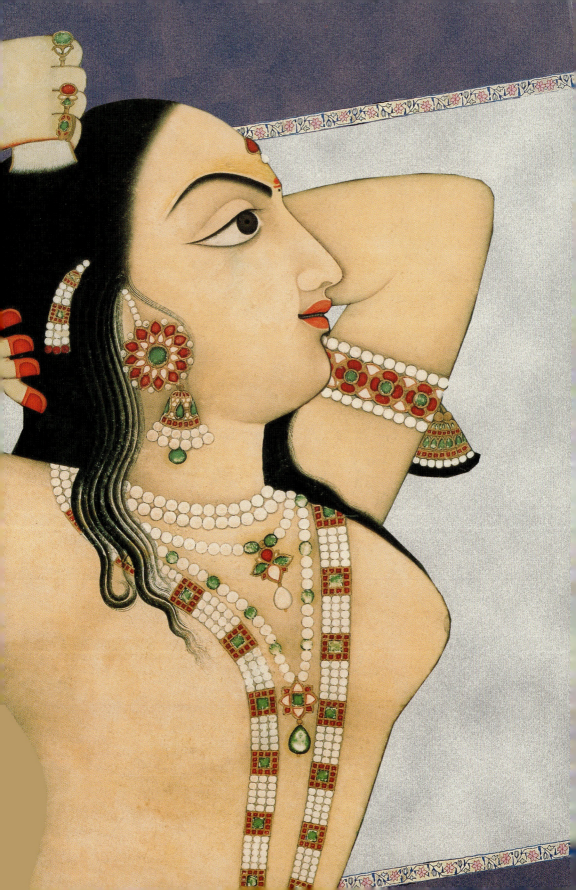

Kama Sutra

✤

Feminine Pleasures

GANESH SAILI

**Lustre Press
Roli Books**

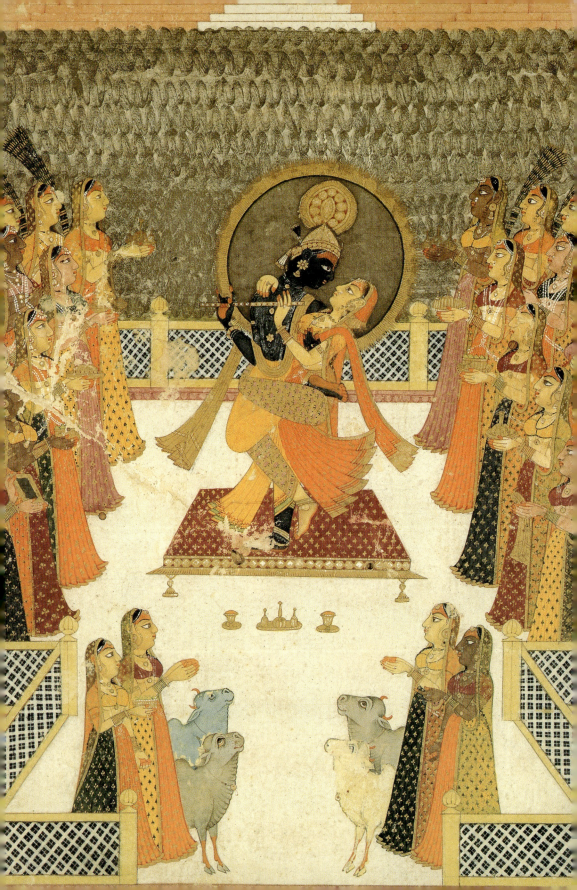

Dedication

This book is written for Abha.
Since the last four decades,
she continues to bear out the adage:
Age cannot wither,
nor custom stale her infinite variety.

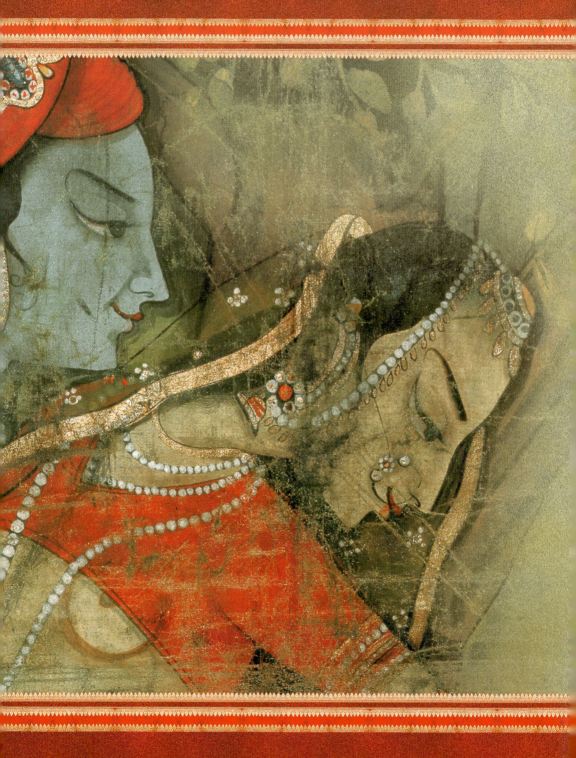

Contents

9
Introduction:
The Feminine in the *Kama Sutra*

25
The Right Balance

41
The Maiden and the Bride

69
Adorning the Body and the Mind

83
The Man and the Woman

97
Love and Art

141
Play of Passion

195
Conclusion:
Towards Eternal Bliss

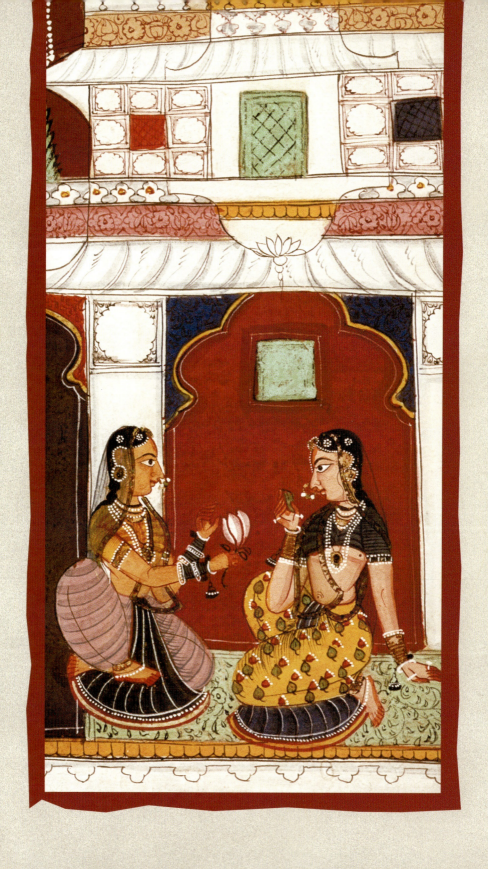

Introduction: The Feminine in the Kama Sutra

If one could willfully enter a time machine to travel back two thousand years in time, to the banks of the holy river Ganges in Benares, one would surely chance upon the Hindu sage Vatsyayana, engaged in codifying human relationships. One would suddenly be in what passes for the oldest living city in the world today—for we have been told that the place is 'older than history, older than legend, older than tradition, and looks twice as old as all of them put together'.

The Hindu sage, Mallinga Vatsyayana, was a compiler and author. He compiled one of the most famous treatise on the art and science of love, the *Kama Sutra*, as part of his religious duties. His sources were the vast body of Hindu erotic treatises already compiled by the first century AD, but the *Kama Sutra* was a watershed in this genre of writing, and bore the mark of the old sage's personality, wisdom and wit.

The Hindu sage had before him the ancient tradition of the philosophy of pleasure, beginning with Kamadeva, the Hindu God of Love, and the first-born of the gods. He is the youngest too for he is born again every day in the meeting and mating of

The Kama Sutra is a treatise on the philosophy of pleasure, compiled by Vatsyayana as much for men as for women.

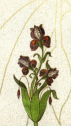

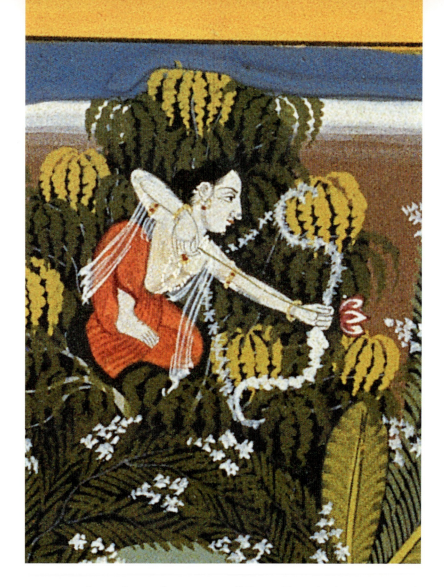

creatures throughout the course of Time. *Kama* is the power and process whereby the one begets oneself as man, beast or plant, and thus carries forward the continued creation of the universe. He does not merely represent sexual pleasure, but all pleasures that arise from the five senses of sound, sight, smell, touch and taste. Anything which appeals to either of these senses individually or cumulatively, can give a man unbounded happiness. It is for this reason, therefore, that six of the original

---

Kamadeva, the God of Love, has as his mate Rati who is the epitome of sensuality.

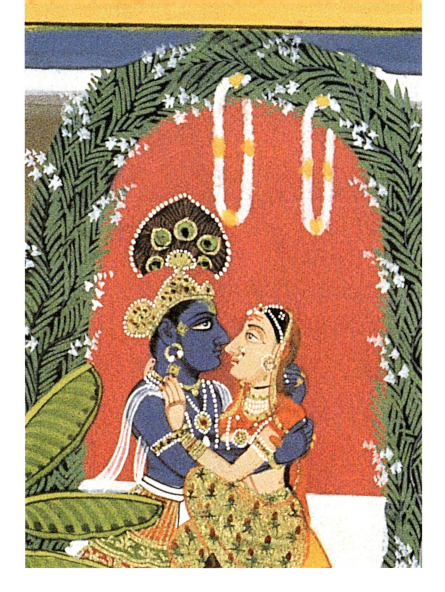

seven chapters of the *Kama Sutra* deal with the conduct of a person in society.

Kamadeva is a brilliant youth, who has by his side, his glamorous mate Rati, all 'lust and sensual delight'. Leading his armoury is *Vasanta* or Spring who with a fragrant wind from the south brings the landscape to bloom and softens all creatures for the sweet, piercing, irresistible onslaught of the God of Love.

The four irresistible instruments of the invincible God of Love

No one can escape the irresistable onslaught of the God of Love, especially in spring.

are a bow entwined with flowers; five arrows whose points are fragrant blossoms; the noose and the hook. These spellbinding weapons he uses to trigger love and induce surrender.

In Hindu mythology, Tvashtri, the Artisan God, created women and it is described thus:

> He took the lightness of the leaf and grace of the fawn, the gaiety of the sun's rays and the tears of mist, the inconstancy of the wind and the timidity of the hare, the vanity of the peacock and the softness of the throat of the swallow. He added the harshness of the diamond, the sweet flavour of honey, the cruelty of the tiger, the warmth of fire and the chill of snow. To this he added the cooing of the dove and the chatter of the jay. He melted all this and formed a woman.

And often, the reader will find her again in the avatar of a lovelorn Radha, alternating between agony and ecstasy, awaiting her beloved at dusk as dark clouds gather across the sky and a parched and panting earth waits for the elusive yet promising rain.

Vatsyayana knew that female sexuality was not something either to be taken for granted or be overlooked. After all, men and women belong to the same species and should so seek the same degree pleasure. It is imperative therefore that women

---

Facing page: It was the duty of a man and a woman to experience love.

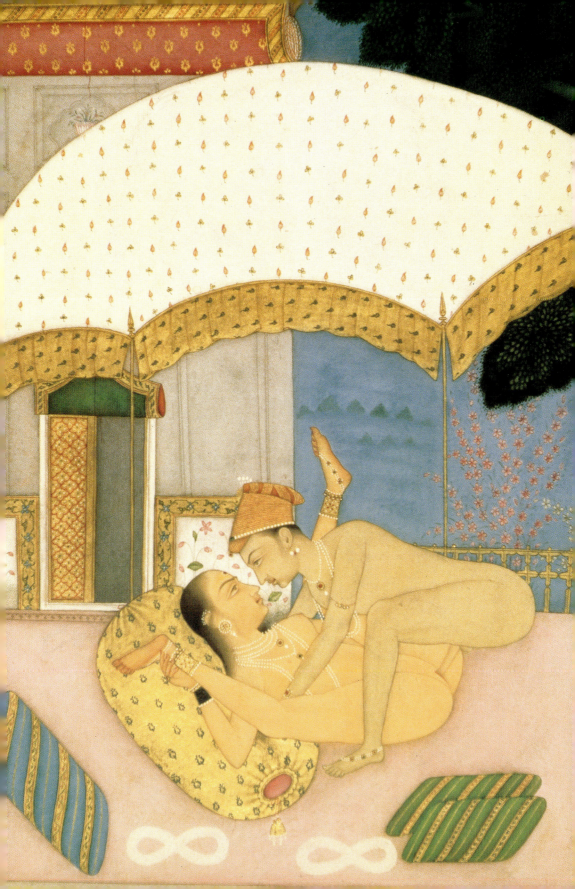

should be as well versed in the art of love as defined and prescribed by the *Kama Sutra*. Vatsyayana admonishes the male of our species:

> Place your pleasures second to hers.

Of course, what amazes the modern reader is that almost two thousand years ago, someone had the ability to understand the fact that sexuality was not and still isn't, the exclusive preserve of just men. So, Rati is the very embodiment of female sexuality and the *Kama Sutra* leaves an equal opportunity for pleasure for both sexes where there are no power games between the male and the female. The sage reminds us:

> Men look for love, women too look for love: women play the main role in the act of intercourse.

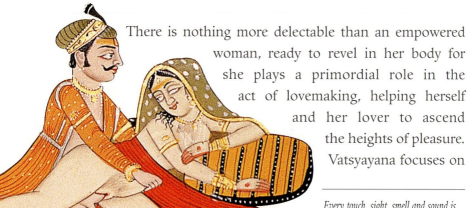

There is nothing more delectable than an empowered woman, ready to revel in her body for she plays a primordial role in the act of lovemaking, helping herself and her lover to ascend the heights of pleasure. Vatsyayana focuses on

Every touch, sight, smell and sound is an erotic moment.

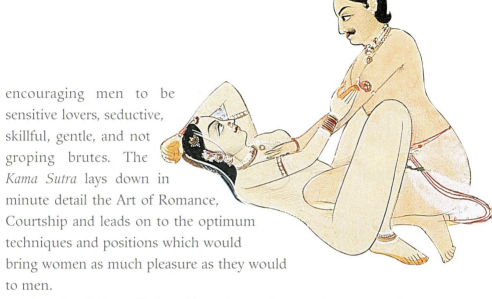

encouraging men to be sensitive lovers, seductive, skillful, gentle, and not groping brutes. The *Kama Sutra* lays down in minute detail the Art of Romance, Courtship and leads on to the optimum techniques and positions which would bring women as much pleasure as they would to men.

Knowing fully well that the path to pleasure for men and women were different, and yet converged at a crossroad, Vatsyayana with his scientific temperament, categorized men and women according to their types: a combination of temperament, nature and physical size. Vatsyayana was aware that there is no substitute for true passion. Lovemaking can blossom only when there is generosity between those who are partners in lovemaking and he guides the lover into the world of intimacy and subtlety which many women crave:

> Every lover must reciprocate the beloved's gesture with equal intensity.... If there is no reciprocity, the beloved will feel dejected and consider the lover as a pillar made of stone. This will result in a highly unsatisfactory union. To keep the flame of passion alive, reciprocity is absolutely essential.

Vatsyayana advises men to be gentle lovers.

Vatsyayana also says:

> At all times, the man must carefully observe every action of the woman he loves, and so gauge her passion and preferences, and act accordingly, to give her the greatest pleasure.

Through the ages, the *Kama Sutra* has taught the novice and the man the numerous ways to make love more sensuously, while instructing woman on how to ignite the flames of desire. The treatise is equally valid today for the 'liberated' modern man and woman. Its message to the world is: 'Happiness and sexual equality belong to every human being,' and still remains one of the earliest attempts to define the wholesome nature of the relationship between a man and a woman, with disarming sexual frankness and candour, defining the many ways in which one can achieve sexual fulfillment while keeping your partner happy.' And even when lovers disagree, we are assured that 'Lovers quarrels are but a renewal of love.'

Believing that the body was a temple, as sacred as the human spirit, the ancients composed scriptures in which they described the quality of life and drew up a catalogue of ways to derive pleasure from the most intimate and natural human activity—sex. The essence of these compilations was that it is the duty of a man and woman to experience love and passion. The ancients knew it

---

Facing page: Sexuality is as much about the body as the mind.

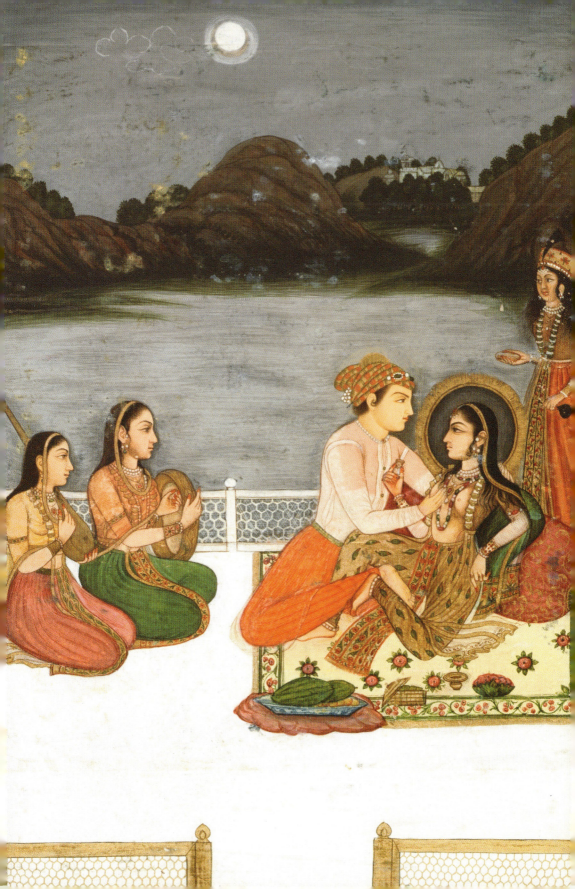

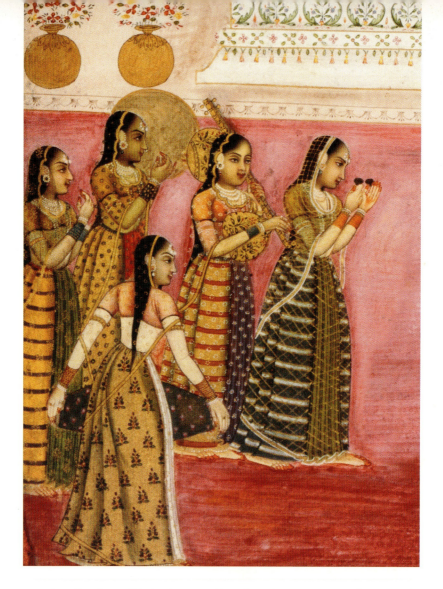

was 'meritorious if it is done well and with the aim to please both participants, and for them to derive pleasure'.

Sexuality in itself is much more than an act of intercourse. The moment eyes meet, hands touch, lips kiss, the breath is felt against the naked skin—every touch, sight, smell and sound is an emotionally charged erotic moment to be savoured and cherished, and seen as the very essence of desire, for without eroticism, the

A woman was expected to be proficient in the art of singing and dancing in order to win over the heart and mind of a man.

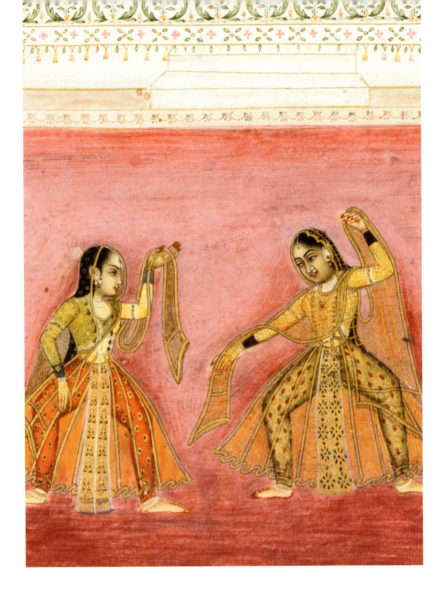

physicality of sex is considered empty. For we are talking about a game whose very aim is pleasure, above all, mutual pleasure.

What then are the ways in which desire is fanned? How do you set up a tryst? Which friends do you use as go-betweens? What perfumes do you use? What do you wear and what do you eat? These are some of the questions that are addressed in the *Kama Sutra*. In the answers lies an unhindered celebration of the female sexuality.

The first quality that the sensuous woman must imbibe is self-respect, and then she must learn to take meticulous care of her

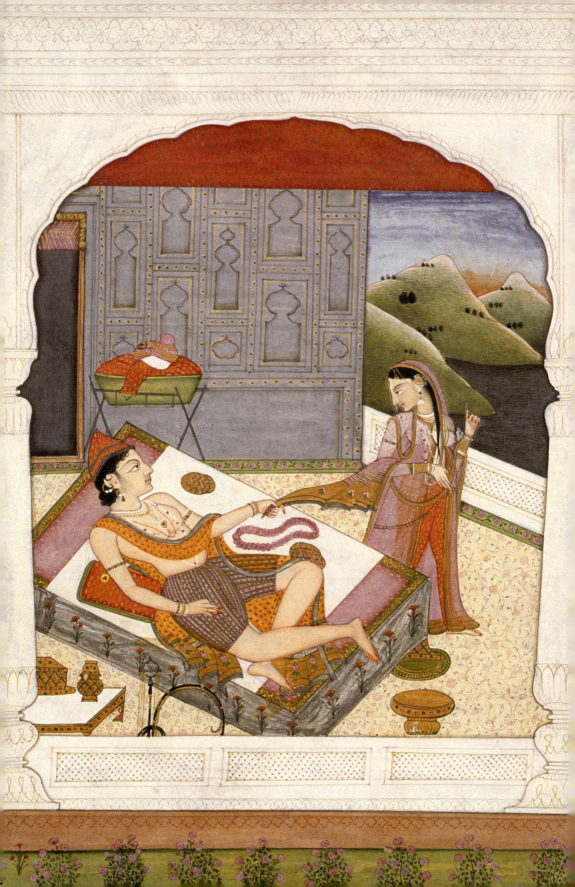

body. Add to these good looks, a happy youth and a liberal attitude and one has what it takes to attract men like moths to a flame. If for some reason, one falls short of some of these qualities, then one could try out the suggestions Vatsyayana gives on beauty care, cosmetics, clothing, perfume, ornaments and attitude.

The *Kama Sutra* also includes the lore of charms, spells, and love-philters. It covers within its ambit the whole range of possible experiences within the sphere of sex, sensual gratification, delight, wish, desire, carnal gratification, lust, love and affection. And the principal aim is to make a success of one's love life. The list of concerns, largely woman-centric, gives us an idea about relationships in those times: for successful conception and childbirth, to win and secure a woman's love, to get a husband for a woman, to recover virility, to beget sons, to counter premature birth, to guard against jealousy, to ensure matrimonial bliss, to name just a few. In our world today, we have yet to definitively resolve these concerns.

In ancient Indian art, women largely occupied the foreground in painting and sculpture. They were cast as goddess, mother and mistress, all at the same time. In the Shashtras, an accomplished woman is described as follows:

> In duty a well-trained servant, in advice as wise as a prince's councillor, in appearance like Lakshmi the Goddess of

---

Facing page: A woman needs to master the codes of social interaction before entering into a relationship with a man.

Wealth, in bad times prudent, in affection like a mother, and in bed, a courtesan!

To be a good lover and a good wife, a woman should know how to sing, strum musical instruments, dance, and compose poetry, make flower-arrangements. Wives, courtesans and young girls were advised to understand the codes of social behaviour before becoming involved with a man. These included:

Guessing peoples thoughts, expressing love, revealing acceptance through body postures, allowing intimacy, love scratches, nibbling gently and seduction, ensuring pleasure for both and playful teasing in moments of intimacy.

The *Kama Sutra* especially guides women through the minefield of human relationships. It begins with how to entice men, reject them gently, please them and in the ultimate analysis change them. Ultimately, sex is not just a habit; it requires constant attention so that it does not lose its charm and importance to become a mere necessity or a banality. And it is the total absence of any notion of sexual guilt or sin that is perhaps the most

---

Elegance and grace were two of the most desirable qualities in the perfect woman.

important message the modern reader can imbibe from the *Kama Sutra,* firmly entrenched today in popular vocabulary and imagination.

Despite being the most famous treatise on sex ever written, rather ironically, only the second part of Sir Richard Burton's translation —which deals exclusively with the famous sixty-four positions —has become synonymous with the *Kama Sutra* of the popular imagination. There is, however, much more to the treatise than that. Sir Richard Burton and his colleagues in the Kama Shastra Society published the *Kama Sutra* in 1883. But for more than half a century this translation remained in an exclusive circle of scholars, bibliophiles and gentlemen with a taste for the exotic. Only a chosen few knew of the existence of the classic. It was only in the 1960s, that the knowledge of the *Kama Sutra* was revealed to the world at large, and it became popular.

Elderly women and friends were always around to help out a neophyte in love.

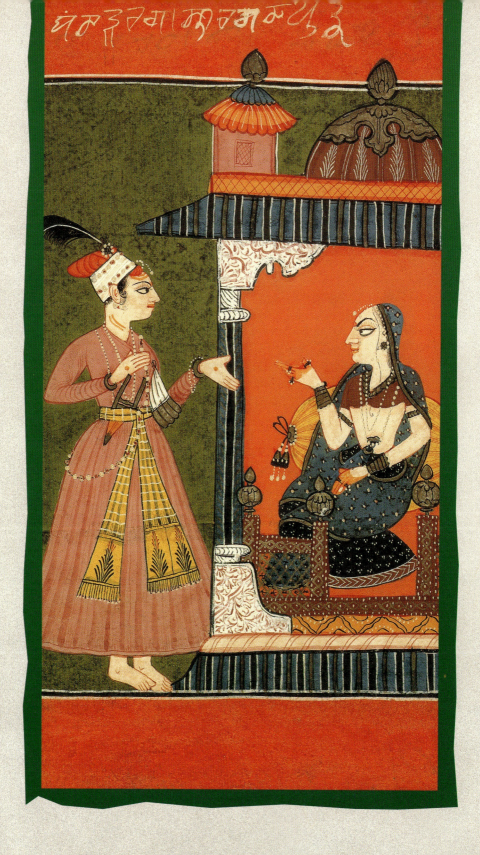

The Right Balance

The *Kama Sutra* is generally regarded as a sex manual. This popular perception of the manual is not only inadequate, but misleading as well. The *Kama Sutra* is not and must not be seen as a book about just the famous 'sixty-four'. Vatsyayana was conscious of the gravity of his task, and wrote:

> This book is not to be used merely as an instrument for the satisfaction of our desires. A person acquainted with the true principles of this science, which preserves his virtue *(dharma),* his wealth *(artha)* and his sensual pleasures *(kama),* and who has regard for the customs of the people, is sure to obtain mastery over his senses. In short, an intelligent and knowing person, attending to *dharma, artha,* and *kama,* without becoming a slave of his passions, will obtain success in everything he may do.

In the ultimate analysis, the subtle arts of sexuality, the body's rapture cannot ever be divorced from the raptures of the soul.

Facing page: The most successful relationship between a man ond a woman is founded on the right balance between virtue, wealth and sensual pleasures.

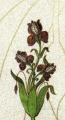

According to the Vedic tradition, human beings are governed by a four-fold structure: *artha* or external security and contentment; *kama* or fulfillment of desires; *dharma* or leading life according to natural laws; *moksha* or evolution towards ultimate freedom.

Vatsyayana believed that a man needed to study the *Kama Sutra* and the arts and sciences subordinate to it, in addition to the study of the arts and sciences of *dharma* and *artha*. A man was to devote his childhood to acquiring learning, his youth and his middle age attending to *artha* and *kama*, and his old age in performing *dharma*, in order to gain *moksha* or release from further transmigration of his soul. The study of *kama,* the enjoyment of appropriate objects with the help of the five senses—touch, smell, sight, sound, taste—provided a man the means and ways of enjoying his life to its fullest extent within the prescribed social and sexual parameters. Following the tenets of *artha* equipped him with the means to achieve, righteously, a comfortable live and standing in society. Following the path of *dharma* gave an ultimate sense of purpose to his existence—attaining liberation from the cycle of death and rebirth.

He believed that human life was precious because only human beings had self-awareness and the potential to realize the Higher Consciousness. So the quest to seek union with the Higher Consciousness was seen as the fundamental purpose of human life. The scriptures therefore recommended that a man should attempt to live on various planes and that he should neither

---

Facing page: A human being must indulge in the pleasures of the senses before attaining the Higher Consciousness.

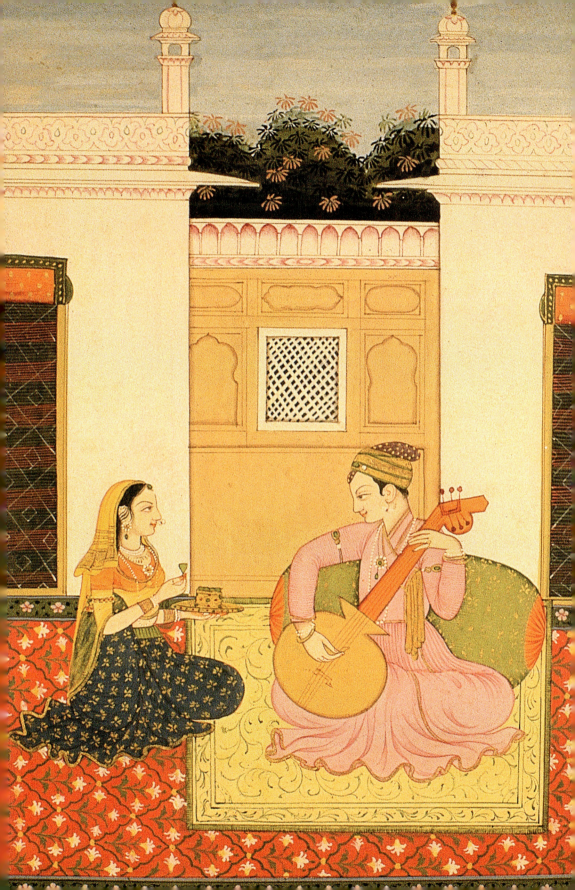

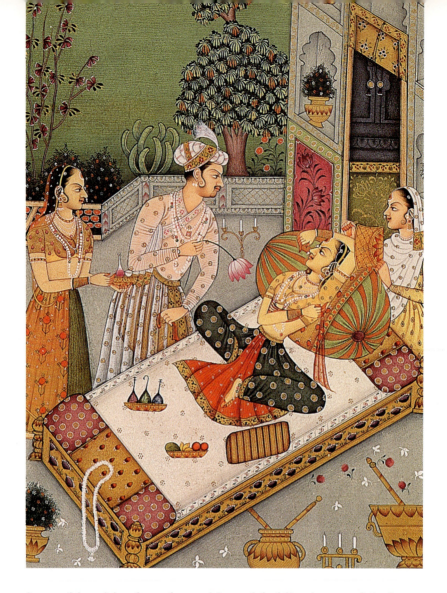

ignore his spiritual needs nor his social obligations and duties to family, community and career. Nor should he ignore his sensuality, his need for love and erotic fulfilment. Vatsyayana's vision of balance was based on this wholeness, an all encompassing ideal where every situation provided an opportunity to become more self-aware and helped in expanding one's capacities. Nor was this learning confined to the physical act, rather it included even the environment, location, behaviour,

---

A woman being tender of nature needs to be wooed with utmost care.

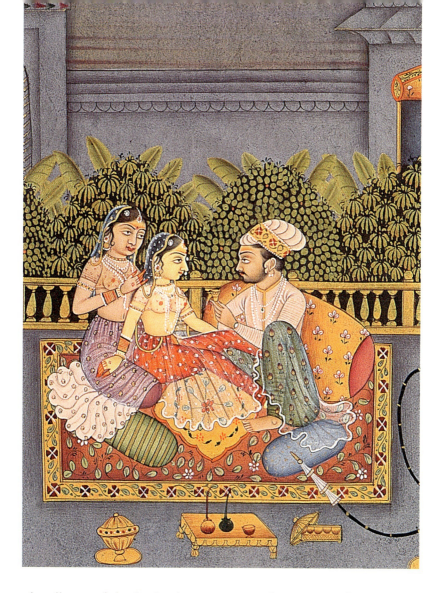

cleanliness of the body, decorousness of manners, allurement, a knowledge of all the arts, a fine sense of aesthetics—all of which came together to work miracles.

Kama was to be learnt from the *Kama Sutra* or aphorisms of love, and from the practice of citizens. And the dissemination of its knowledge was not to be restricted only to men. Vatsyayana suggested that before marriage young maids too were to study the *Kama Sutra* along with its arts and sciences which include

Partners in love need to go beyond the physical to attain a higher spiritual bliss.

everything from making artificial flowers and playing on musical glasses filled with water, to knowledge of mines and quarries, and even warfare. Once married, they were to continue studying the *Kama Sutra* with the consent of their husbands. While many learned men objected to women studying any of the sciences, including the *Kama Sutra*, Vatsyayana was of the opinion:

> If a wife becomes separated from her husband, and falls into distress, she can support herself easily, even in a foreign country, by means of her knowledge of these arts.

Even a sketchy knowledge of these sciences empowered a woman to fend for herself, although the putting to practice of such knowledge would be largely dependant on circumstances. But a woman needed to be as well versed in the sciences for reasons that went beyond those of mere survival. They were to be equal partners in the game of love. A man well versed in the sciences and arts, very soon gained the hearts of

This and facing page: The ideal household should be surrounded by a garden.

women, despite being acquainted with them only for a short time. And if he was skilled in the arts, a poet, a marvellous storyteller, an eloquent man, possessed of a great mind, energetic, a visionary, perseverant, devoted, free from anger, liberal, affectionate to parents, sociable, skilled in completing verses begun by others, a sportsperson, healthy, strong, brave, not addicted to drinking, with sexual prowess, respectful to women, wealthy, free from envy, and lastly free from suspicion—he had the makings of a fine man and an apt householder.

The ideal abode for the householder would be:

> ... a house in a city, or a large village, or in the vicinity of good men or in a place which is the resort of many persons. This abode should be situated near some water, and divided into different compartments for different purposes. It should be surrounded by a garden, and also contain two rooms, an outer and an inner one. The inner room should be occupied by the women, while the outer room, balmy with rich perfumes,

---

Following pages 32-33: Harmony in a household depends largely on the gentle nature of the woman.

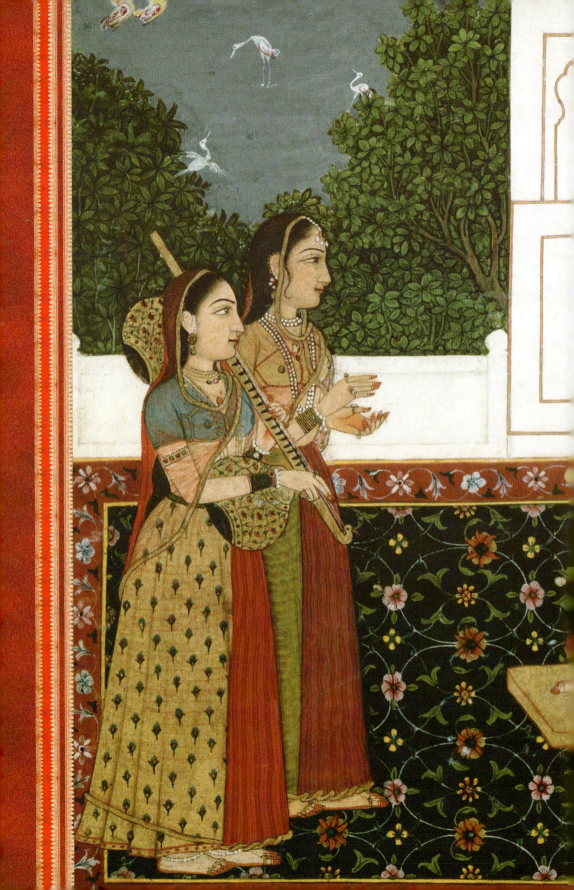

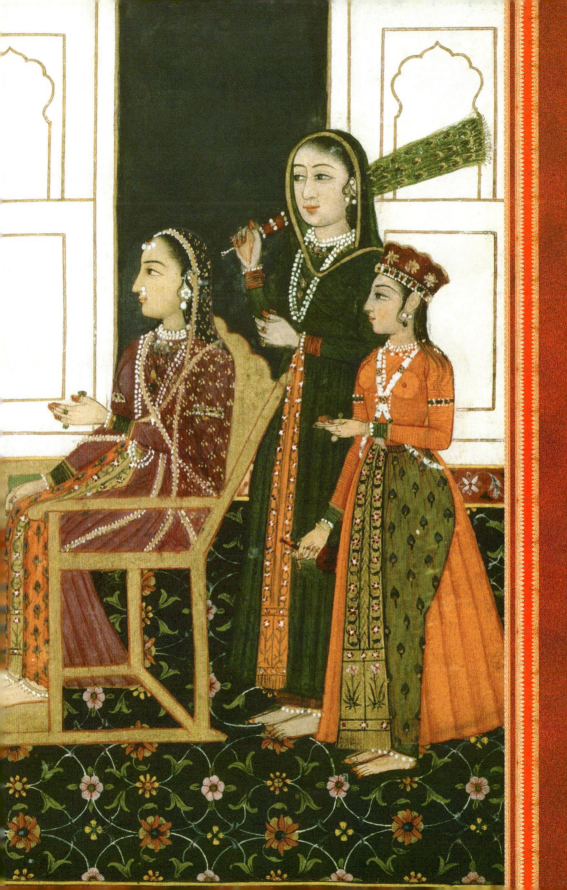

should contain a bed, soft, agreeable to the sight, covered with a clean white cloth, low in the middle part, having garlands and bunches of flowers upon it, and a canopy above it, and two pillows, one at the top, another at the bottom. There should be also a sort of couch besides and at the head of this a sort of stool, on which should be placed the fragrant ointments for the night, as well as flowers, pots containing collyrium and other fragrant substances, things used for perfuming the mouth, and the bark of the common citron tree. Near the couch, on the ground, there should be a pot for spitting, a box containing ornaments, and also a lute hanging from a peg made of the tooth of an elephant, a board for drawing, a pot containing perfume, some books, and some garlands of the yellow amaranth flowers. Not far from the couch and on the ground, there should be a round seat, a toy cart, and a board for playing with dice; outside the outer room there should be cases of birds and a separate place for spinning, carving and such like diversions. In the garden there should be a whirling swing and a common swing, as also a bower of creepers covered with flowers, in which a raised parterre should be made for sitting.

This detailed description of the householder's abode gently refers to an inner room for women—subtly alluding to the ideal woman of the house: beautiful, amenable, with a good body, ready to

---

Facing page: A clean beautiful house resounding with birdsong sets the mood for love.

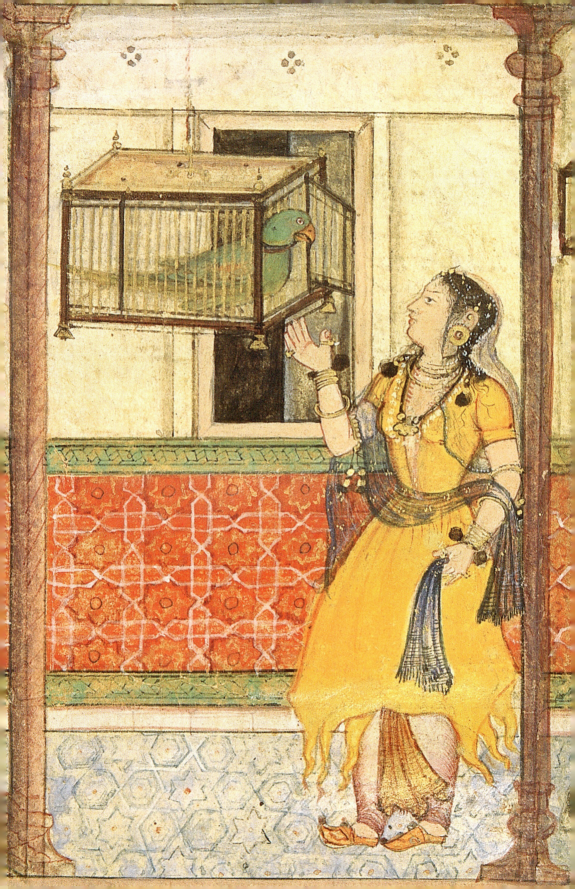

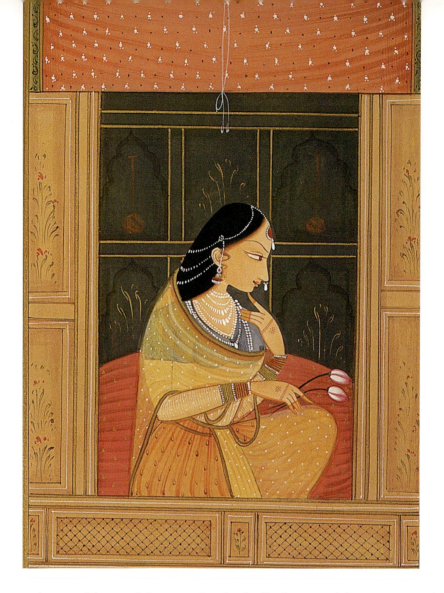

enjoy wealth; participate enthusiastically in sexual intercourse; have the same desires as her man; knowledgeable and interested in educating herself, free from greed, sociable and interested in the arts; intelligent, of good disposition and good manners; and straightforward in her behaviour. Women who were loud, mean, laughed loudly, malicious, angry, avaricious, dull, slothful and stupid were to be avoided. Once the woman became a wife, her conduct and behaviour had to be exemplary.

A woman's physical beauty should be the reflection of a beautiful mind.

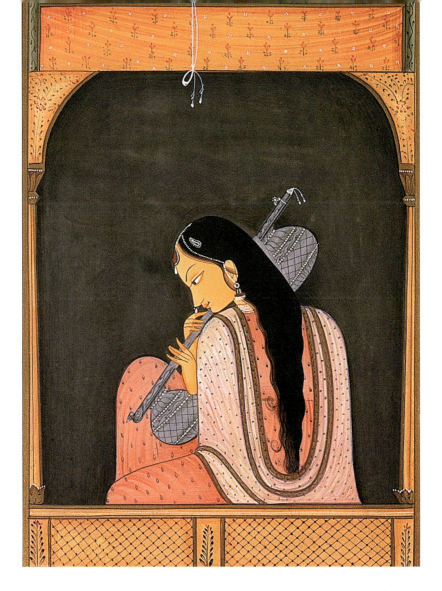

A typical day in the life of a householder unfolded as follows:

Now the householder, having got up in the morning and performed his necessary duties, should wash his teeth, apply a limited quantity of ointments and perfumes to his body, put some ornaments on his person and collyrium on his eyelids and below his eyes, colour his lips with alacktaka, and look at himself in the glass. Having then eaten betel leaves,

A woman accomplished in the sixty-four arts is the pride and joy of her lover.

with other things that give fragrance to the mouth, he should perform his usual business. He should bathe daily, anoint his body with oil every other day, apply a lathering substance to his body every three days, get his head (including face) shaved every four days, and the other parts of his body every five or ten days. All these things should be done without fail, and the sweat of the armpits should also be removed. Meals should be taken in the forenoon, in the afternoon and again at night.... After breakfast, parrots and other birds should be taught to speak, and the fighting of cocks, quails, and rams should follow. A limited time should be devoted to diversions with *pithamardas* (confidantes), *vitas* (parasites) and *vidushakas* (jesters) and then should be taken the midday sleep. After this the householder, having put on his clothes and ornaments, should, during the afternoon, converse with his friends. In the evening there should be singing, and after that the householder, along with his friend, should await in

---

Before meeting her husband, a woman is to adorn herself with jewellery and beautiful clothes, and wear perfume.

his room, previously decorated and perfumed, the arrival of the woman that may be attached to him, or he may send a female messenger for her, or go to her himself. After her arrival at his house, he and his friend should welcome her, and entertain her with a loving and agreeable conversation. Thus end the duties of the day.

When the wife meets her husband, she is always to be well dressed, adorned with jewellery and flowers and be perfumed with sweet-smelling ointments or scents. She is required to observe the necessary rituals, fasts and vows for her husband. She should be a careful housekeeper, stocking up on commodities during different times of the year when these are cheap and be careful with money. She should neither disclose nor talk about her husband's wealth and be discreet about the secrets that she shares with her husband. She should strive to surpass other women of her own rank with her intelligence, appearance, her competence as a cook, her demeanour and in the service of her husband. She should be sociable, welcome her husband's friends and be respectful to her in-laws. Women who are vain, too self-absorbed, greedy, loud and disrespectful are to be avoided.

Vatsyayana's protagonists would have more contemporary faces today. In our times, one need not necessarily equate 'householders' with people who are married to each other. The scale and range of emotions people in love go through remain almost the same, within and beyond the pale of marriage.

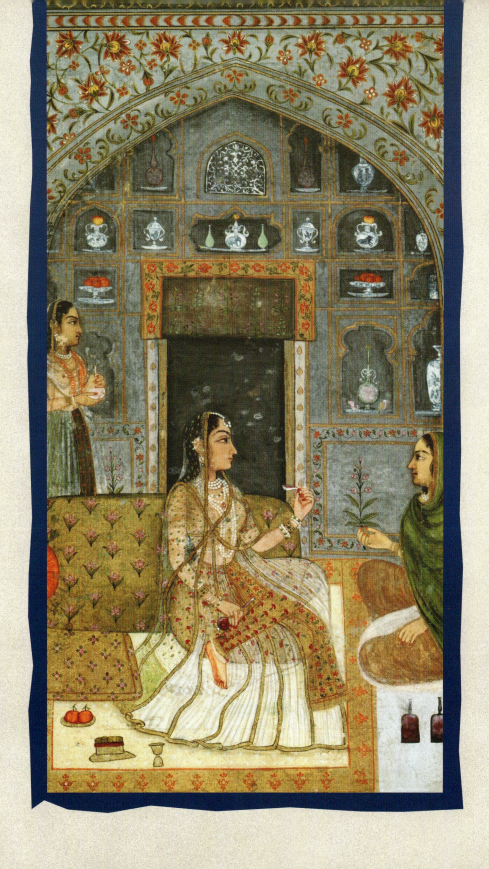

The Maiden and the Bride

Young maidens were encouraged to study the subject of *kama* along with its arts and sciences before marriage. Vatsyayana was of opinion that since women anyway knew and learnt about sex through personal experience, their studying it was imperative not just as the practice of a science but in order to understand and gain mastery over the rules and laws on which this science was based. According to the *Kama Sutra*:

> When a girl becomes marriageable, her parents should dress her smartly, and should place her where she can be easily seen by all. Every afternoon, having dressed her and decorated her in a becoming manner, they should send her with her female companions to sports, sacrifices, and marriage ceremonies, and thus show her to advantage in society. They should also receive with kind words and signs of friendliness those of an auspicious appearance who may come accompanied by their friends and relations for the purpose of marrying their daughter, and under some pretext or other having first dressed her becomingly, should then present her to them. After this they should await the

Facing page: Before marriage, girls were encouraged to study the Kama Sutra *in detail.*

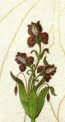

pleasure of fortune, and with this object should appoint a future day on which a determination could be come to with regard to their daughter's marriage. On this occasion, when the persons have come, the parents of the girl should ask them to bathe and dine, and should say, 'Everything will take place at the proper time,' and should not then comply with the request but should settle the matter later.

Vatsyayana further elaborates on the notion of compatibility and the befitting connection between partners:

That should be known as a high connection when a man, after marrying a girl, has to serve her and her relations afterwards like a servant, and such a connection is censured by the good. On the other hand, that reproachable connection, where a man together with his relations, lords it over his wife, is called a low connection by the wise. But when both the man and the woman afford mutual pleasure to each other, and where the relatives on both sides pay respect to one another, such is called a connection in the proper sense of the word. Therefore men should contract neither a high connection by which he is obliged to bow down afterwards to his kinsmen, nor a low connection, which is universally reprehended by all.

Facing page: The Kama Sutra *lays great emphasis on the physical and mental compatibility of partners.*

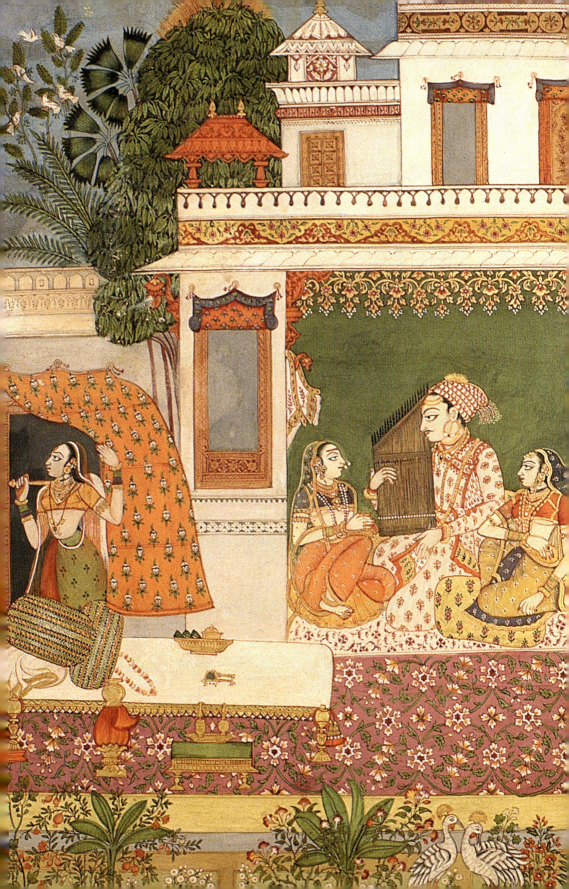

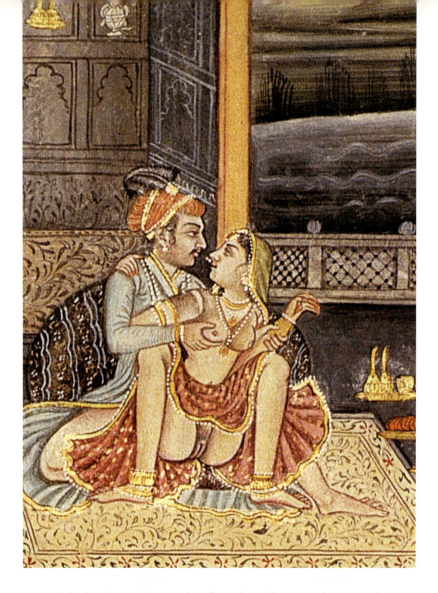

A girl who is much sought after should marry the man that she likes, and whom she thinks would be obedient to her, and capable of giving her pleasure. But when from the desire of wealth a girl is married by her parents to a rich man without taking into consideration the character or looks of the bridegroom, or when given to a man who has several wives, she never becomes attached to the man, even though he be endowed with good qualities, obedient to her will,

Vatsyayana strongly advocates fidelity between partners.

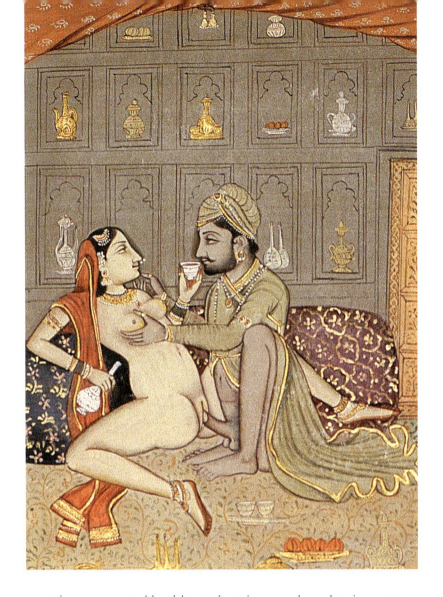

active, strong, and healthy and anxious to please her in every way. A husband, who is obedient but yet master of him, though he is poor and not good looking, is better than one, who is common to many women, even though he be handsome and attractive. The wives of the rich, where there are many wives, are not generally attached to their husbands, and are not confidential with them, and even though they possess all the external enjoyments of life, still

Partners in love need to be able to confide in each other.

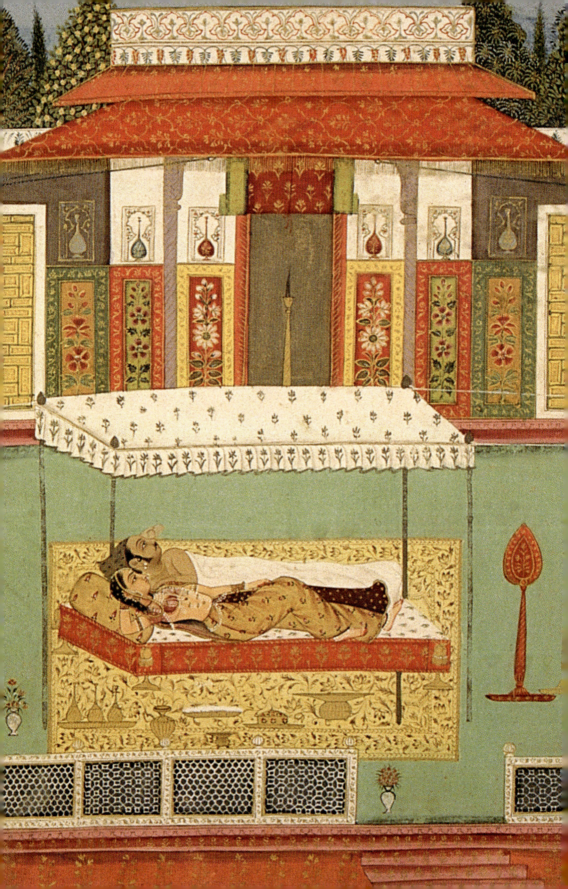

have recourse to other men. A man who is of a low mind, who has fallen from his social position, and who is much given to travelling, does not deserve to be married; neither does one who has many wives and children, or one who is devoted to sport and gambling and who comes to his wife only when he likes.

But Vatsyayana was ahead of his times in affirming that of all the lovers of a girl:

> ... he only is her true husband who possesses the qualities that are liked by her, and only such a husband really enjoys true superiority over her, because he is the husband of love.

Vatsyayana leads us from the choice of the right groom, to the right etiquette to be followed between a couple immediately after marriage:

> For the first three days after marriage, the girl and her husband should sleep on the floor, abstain from sexual pleasures, and eat their food without seasoning it either with alkali or salt. For the next seven days they should bathe amidst the sounds of auspicious musical instruments, should decorate themselves, dine together, and pay attention to their relations as well as to those who may have

Facing page: Newly married couples must get to know each other a bit before indulging in the final act of love.

come to witness their marriage… . On the night of the tenth day the man should begin in a lonely place with soft words, and thus create confidence in the girl. There are some authors who say that for the purpose of winning her over he should not speak to her for three days.

Many feel that if the man does not speak with his newly wed bride for long time, she may becoming dejected, and begin to despise him. Vatsyayana does not suggest any delay in winning over her confidence, but he does suggest that the man abstain at first from indulging in sexual pleasures. Women being of a tender nature want tender beginnings, and when men with whom they are but slightly acquainted force them into a situation they may not emotionally or physically be capable of dealing with, sometimes they suddenly end up hating sex and oftentimes, hating males. The man should therefore approach the girl according to her liking, and should make use of those devices by which he may be able to increasingly gain her confidence. These devices include:

He should embrace her first of all in the way she likes most, because it

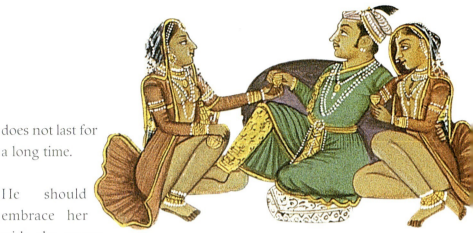

does not last for a long time.

He should embrace her with the upper part of his body, because that is easier and simpler. If the girl is grown up, or if he has known her for some time, he may embrace her by the light of a lamp, but if he is not well acquainted with her, or if she is a young girl, he should then embrace her in darkness.

When the girl accepts the embrace, the man should put a *tambula* or screw of betel nut and betel leaves in her mouth, and if she will not take it, he should induce her to do so by conciliatory words, entreaties, oaths, and kneeling at her feet, for it is a universal rule that however bashful or angry a woman may be, she never disregards a man's kneeling at her feet. At the time of giving this *tambula* he should kiss her mouth softly and gracefully without making any sound. When she is gained over in this respect he should then make her talk, and so that she may be induced to talk he should ask her questions about things of which he knows or pretends to know nothing, and which can be answered in a few words. If she does not speak to him, he should not

This and facing page: A man must never force himself on his newly wed bride, but win her over with love.

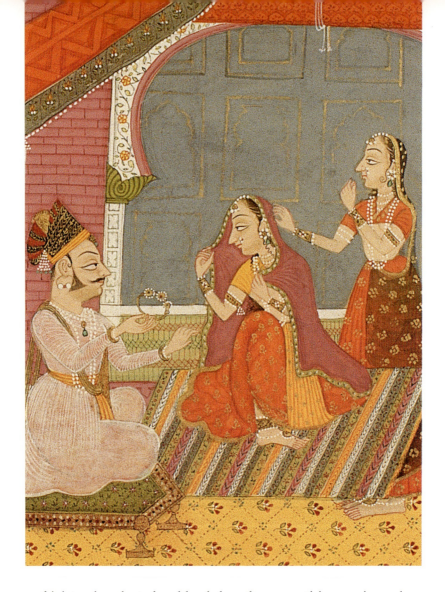

frighten her, but should ask her the same thing again and again in a conciliatory manner. If even then she does not speak, he should urge her to give a reply since, 'All girls hear everything said to them by men, but do not they sometimes say a single word.' When she feels so, the girl should give replies by shakes of the head, but if she has quarrelled with the man she should not even do that. When she is asked whether she wishes for him, and whether she likes him, she

Often, a man needs to seek help from his wife's friends to win over her confidence.

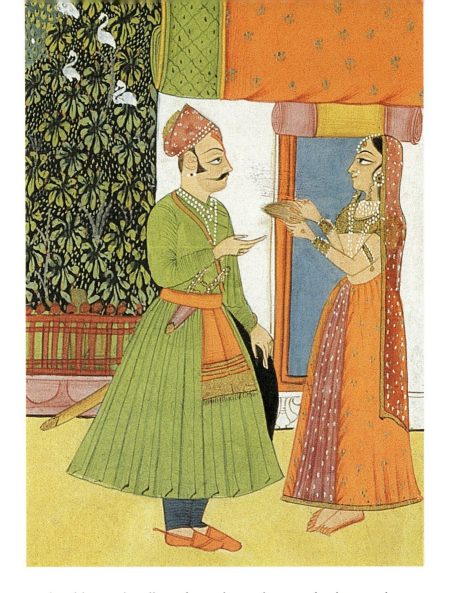

should remain silent for a long time, and when at last cornered to answer, she should give him a favourable reply by just a nod of her head. If the man is previously acquainted with the girl he should converse with her by means of a female friend, who may be favourable to him, and in the confidence of both, and carry on the conversation on both sides. On such an occasion the girl should smile with her head bent down, and if the female

Offering her husband the tambula is a woman's invitation to love.

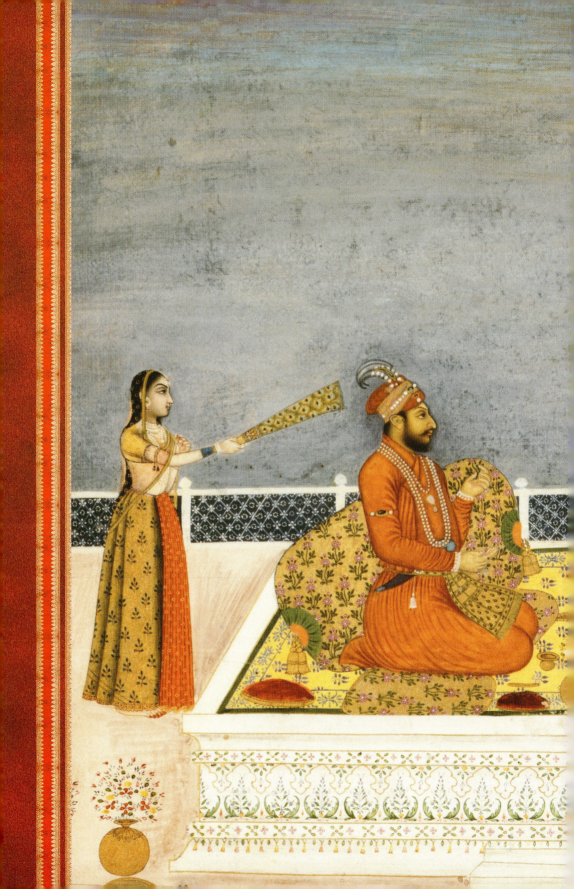

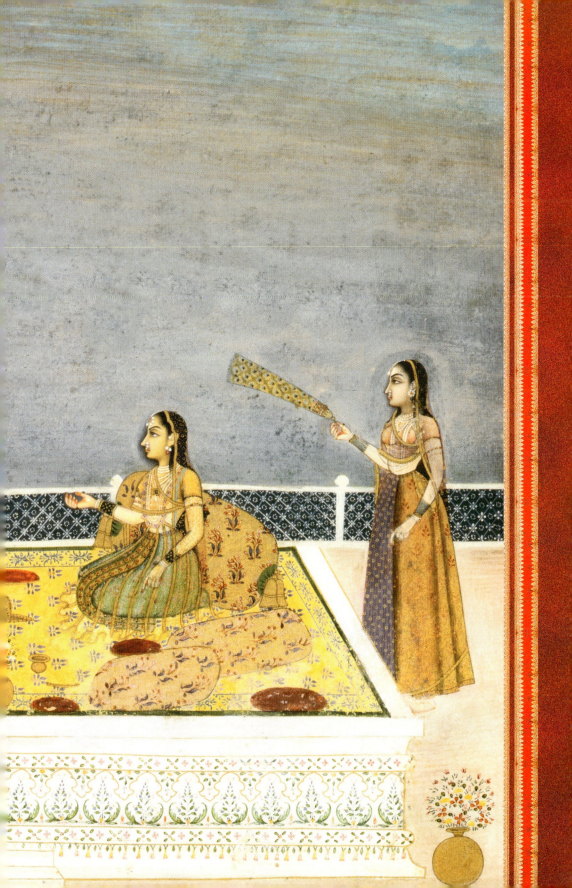

friend says more on her part than she was desired to do, she should chide her and dispute with her. The female friend should say in jest even what she is not desired to say by the girl, and add, 'She says so,' on which the girl should say indistinctly and prettily, 'Oh no! I did not say so,' and she should then smile and throw an occasional glance towards the man.

If the girl is familiar with the man, she should place near him, without saying anything, the *tambula*, the ointment, or the garland that he may have asked for, or she may tie them up in his upper garment. While she is engaged in this, the man should touch her young breasts in the sounding way of pressing with the nails, and if she prevents him doing this he should say to her, 'I will not do it again if you will embrace me,' and should in this way cause her to embrace him. While she is embracing him he should pass his hand repeatedly over and about her body. By and by he should place her in his lap, and try more and more to gain her consent, and if she will not yield to him he should frighten her by saying 'I shall impress marks of my teeth and nails on your lips and breasts, and then make similar marks on my own body, and shall tell my friends that you did them. What will you say then?' In this and other ways, as fear and

---

Preceding pages 52-53: Building up the right atmosphere helps in building up the right rapport between lovers. Facing page: A woman would only yield to love if she is gently led to it.

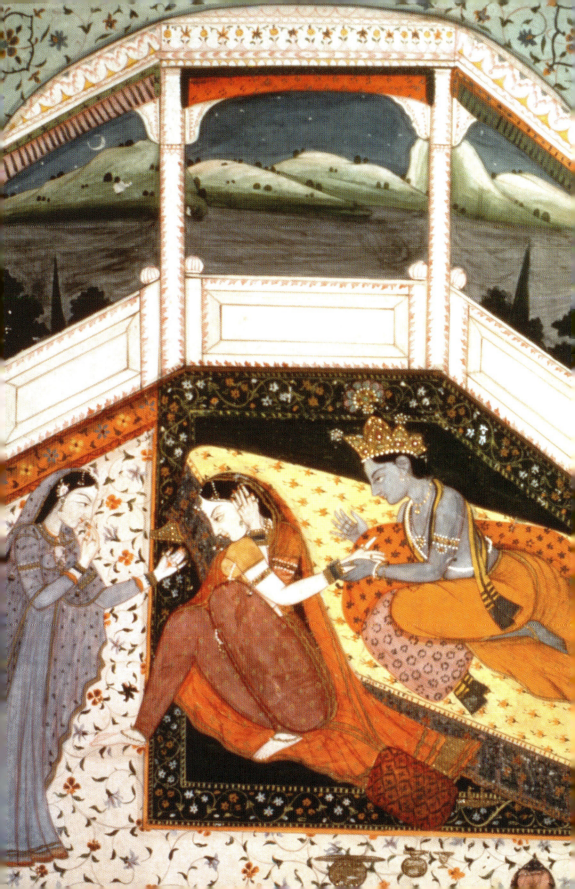

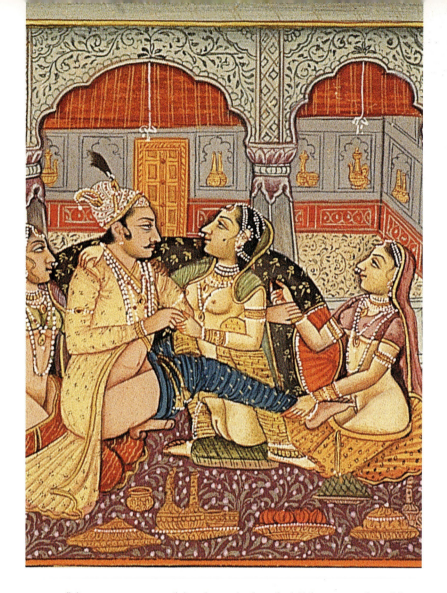

confidence are created in the minds of children, so should he gain her over to his wishes.

On the second and third nights, after her confidence has increased still more, he should feel the whole of her body with his hands, and kiss her all over; he should also place his hands upon her thighs and shampoo them, and if he succeeds in this he should then shampoo the joints of her

Vatsyayana instructs men on the fine art of undressing a woman as a prelude to love.

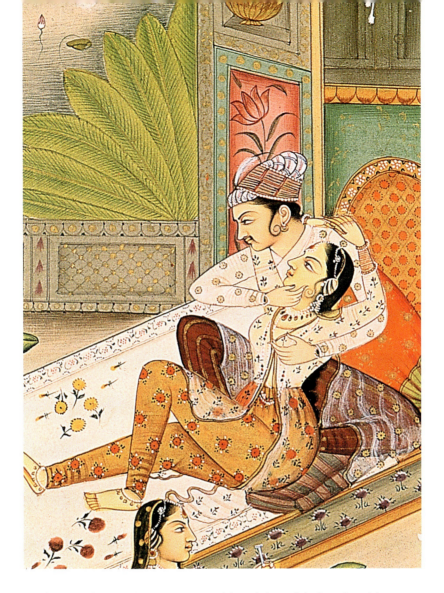

thighs. If she tries to prevent him doing this he should say to her, 'What harm is there in doing it?' and should persuade her to let him do it. After gaining this point he should touch her intimate parts, loosen her girdle and the knot of her dress, and turning up her lower garment should shampoo the joints of her naked thighs. Under various pretences he should do all these things, but he should not at that time begin actual congress. After this he should teach

A subtle look and touch set in motion the wheels of desire.

her the sixty-four arts, should tell her how much he loves her, and describe to her the hopes which he formerly entertained regarding her. He should also promise to be faithful to her in future and should dispel all her fears with respect to rival women, and, at last, after having overcome her bashfulness, he should begin to enjoy her in a way so as not to frighten her.

Often a lingering glance, the flutter of the eyelids, or the unspoken word, carry a far more powerful message of sensuality than the physical act of intercourse. An affectionate touch or a tender caress often speaks louder than words. We often hark back to an era gone by where grace and sensuousness were the mainstay of every relationship, where lovers delighted in the fragrance of jasmine flowers, the melody of songbirds, a touch and the ritual of seduction that presaged lovemaking. The *Kama Sutra* lays great emphasis on mastering the game of wooing with grace and the need to understand the nuances of foreplay as a prelude to sexual gratification—the 'social acceptability' of the relationship notwithstanding.

Foreplay begins with desire in the mind as it contemplates physical intimacy with a loved one. Desire encompasses the building up of stimuli that lead up to orgasm for mutual gratification. Undressing, kissing, petting, flirting, oral sex, cuddling are all-important especially for women who need prolonged stimulation in order to be completely aroused. Ultimately good sex is about attentiveness, being sensitive to the partner's needs and the desire to ensure that the experience is intensely pleasurable and memorable for both.

> A man acting according to the inclinations of a girl should try and gain her over so that she may love him and place her confidence in him. A man does not succeed either by implicitly following the inclination of a girl, or by wholly opposing her, and he should therefore adopt a middle course. He who knows how to make himself beloved by women, as well as to increase their honour and create confidence in them, this man becomes an object of their love. But she despises him, who neglects a girl thinking she is too bashful, as a beast ignorant of the working of the female mind. Moreover, a girl forcibly enjoyed by one who does not understand the hearts of girls becomes nervous, uneasy, and dejected, and suddenly begins to hate the man who has taken advantage of her; and then, when her love is not understood or returned, she sinks into despondency, and becomes either a hater of mankind altogether, or, hating her own man, she has recourse to other men.

The game of love needs to be played by partners who are above all understanding of each other's needs, and respectful of each other as human beings.

Even though Vatsyayana's definition of a 'virtuous wife' reads like an anachronism in our days and times, what he essentially seems to plead for is a stable relationship that is carefully nurtured by the partners:

> A virtuous woman, who has affection for her husband, should act in conformity with his wishes as if he were a divine being, and with his consent should take upon herself the care of his family. She should keep the whole house well cleaned, and arrange flowers of various kinds in different parts of it, and make the floor smooth and polished so as to give the whole a neat and becoming appearance. She should surround the house with a garden, and place ready in it all the materials required for the morning, noon and evening prayers.

> The wife, whether she is a woman of noble family, or a virgin widow remarried, or a concubine should lead a chaste life, devoted to her husband, and doing everything for his welfare. Women acting thus, acquire *dharma*, *artha*, and *kama*, obtain a high position, and generally keep their husbands devoted to them.

A man may, however:

> ... resort to the wife of another, for the purpose of saving his own life, when he perceives that his love for her proceeds from one degree of intensity to another.

Facing page: A woman noble in mind and spirit is whole-heartedly devoted to her partner.

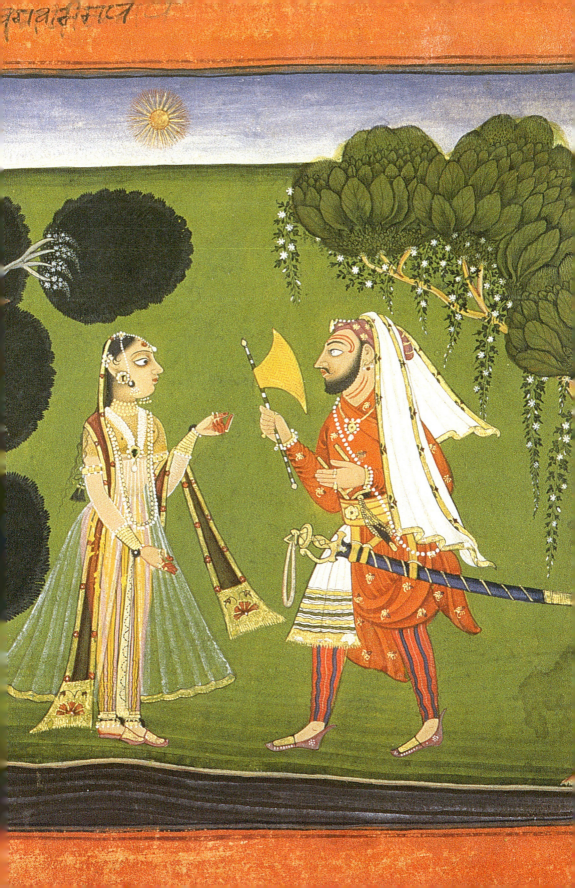

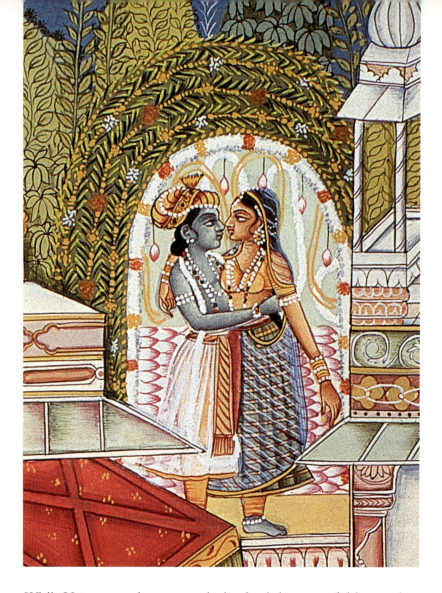

While Vatsyayana does not actively plead the case of this practice, he is prudent enough not turn a blind eye to such a possibility.

These degrees are ten in number, and are distinguished by the following marks:

- ✤ Love of the eye
- ✤ Attachment of the mind
- ✤ Constant reflection

Love between a man and a woman needs constant nurturing.

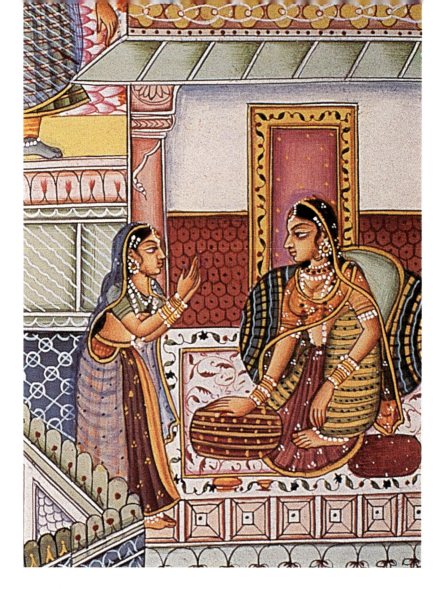

- Destruction of sleep
- Emaciation of the body
- Turning away from objects of enjoyment
- Removal of shame
- Madness
- Fainting
- Death

A prudent woman would heed the advice of those more experienced in love.

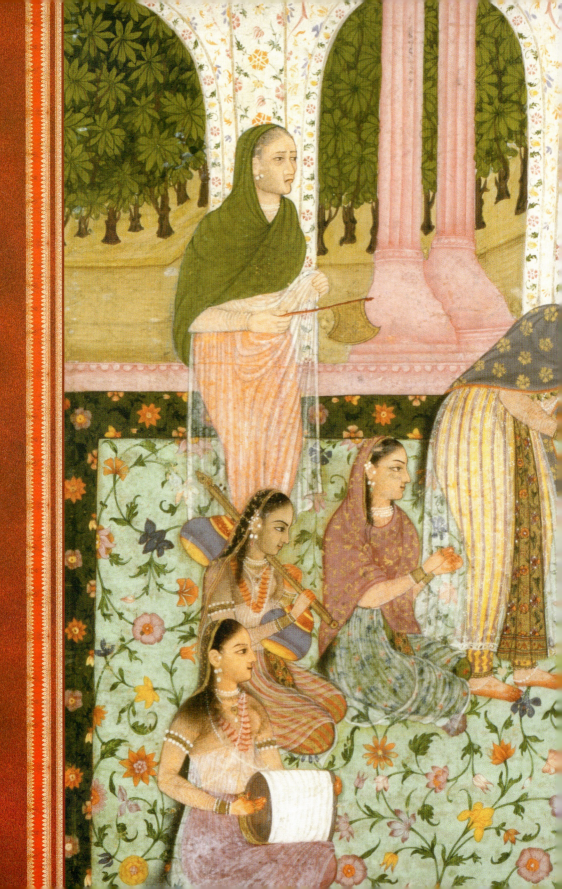

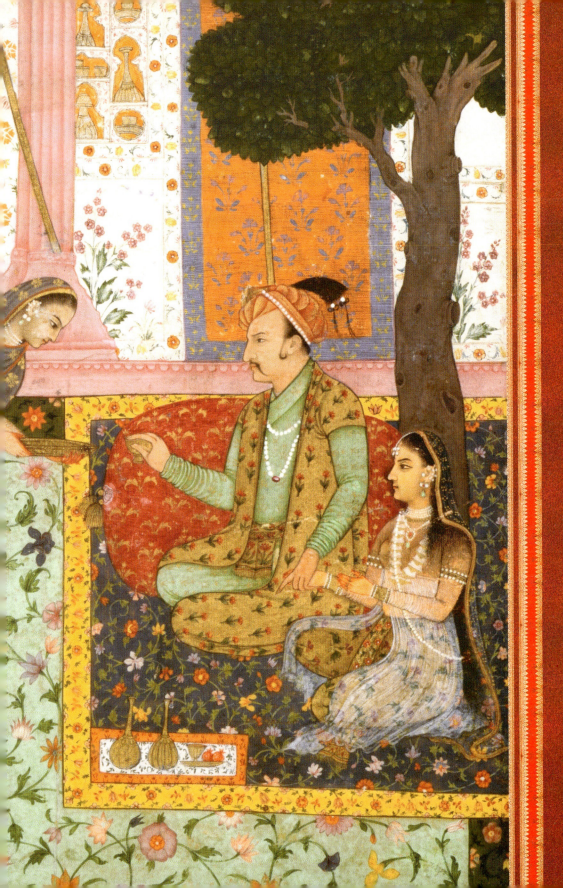

The causes of a woman rejecting the addresses of a man are:
- ♣ Affection for her husband
- ♣ Desire of lawful progeny
- ♣ Want of opportunity
- ♣ Anger at being addressed by the man too familiarly
- ♣ Difference in rank of life
- ♣ Want of certainty on account of the man being devoted to travelling
- ♣ Thinking that the man may be attached to some other person
- ♣ Fear of the man's not keeping his intentions secret
- ♣ Thinking that the man is too devoted to his friends, having too great a regard for them
- ♣ The apprehension that he is not in earnest
- ♣ Bashfulness on account of his being an illustrious man
- ♣ Fear on account of his being powerful, or possessed of too impetuous passion, in the case of the 'deer' woman
- ♣ Bashfulness on account of his being too clever
- ♣ The thought of having once lived with him on friendly terms only
- ♣ Contempt of his want of knowledge of the world
- ♣ Distrust of his low character
- ♣ Disgust at his want of perception of her love for him
- ♣ In the case of an 'elephant' woman, the thought that he is a 'hare' man, or a man weak of passion

Preceding pages 64-65: A man well-versed in the Shastras knows of the pitfalls of seducing other men's wives.
Facing page: Men are attracted to women accomplished in the arts.

- Compassion lest anything should befall him on account of his passion
- Despair at her own imperfections
- Fear of discovery
- Disillusion at seeing his grey hair or shabby appearance
- Fear that he may be employed by her husband to test her chastity
- The thought that he has too much regard to morality

A man who is well versed in the Shastras would know about the ways of winning over the wives of other people, and would never be deceived in the case of his own wives. Vastyayana, however, strongly discourages making use of these ways for seducing the wives of others, because such overtures often result in disasters, and the destruction of *dharma* and *artha*. He reiterates that:

> This book which is intended for the good of the people, and to teach them the ways of guarding their own wives, should not be, made use of merely for gaining over the wives of others.

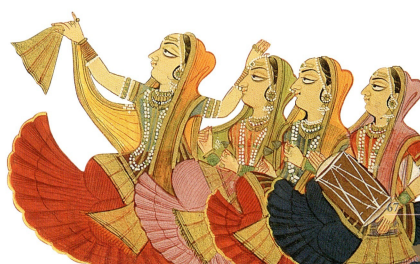

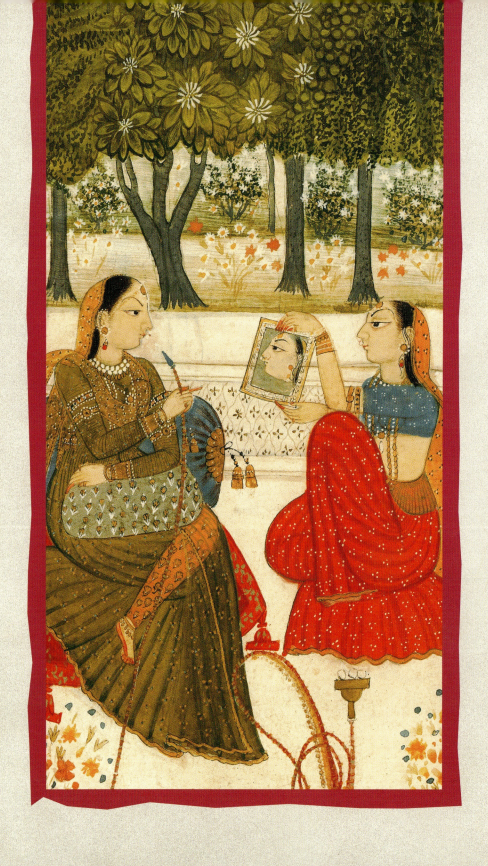

Adorning the Body and the Mind

Ancient texts identify sixteen different embellishments (*solah-shringar*), used to celebrate the beauty and divinity of the female form. Sixteen is a significant number corresponding to the sixteen phases of the moon, which in turn are associated with a woman's menstrual cycle. Thus a young woman of sixteen is considered to be the embodiment of perfection, since she is at the peak of her physical charms. The term *shringar* is associated with Sri, another name for Laksmi, the Goddess of Female beauty, luck, prosperity and fertility who is also venerated as an ideal wife. Women realized the spiritual side of ornamentation and believed that by adorning their bodies, they also satisfied a universal longing for the embellishment of its intangible counterpart: the human spirit.

Thus, women continue to embellish their bodies as a means of expressing their own aesthetic sentiments and to attract men:

❧ NEPATHYAPRAYOGA ❧

Nepathyaprayoga undertakes the study of what we now call couture, that is fashion, fabrics and the art of dressing up to

---

Facing page: Women embellished their bodies as an expression of their own aesthetic concerns.

maximize and enhance one's assets. Since this presupposes a sense of drama, the art of making up for the stage and theatre was also included in this category.

✤ KARNAPATRABHANGA ✤

This has to do with the decoration of the ears. The different types of ornaments like earrings, loops, flowers initially made out of ivory, conch shells, leaves and flowers were replaced with metals like iron and then silver, gold and precious gems. According to some scholars, the art of painting the forehead, over the eyebrows, and other parts of the face up to the ear with sandal paste, vermilion among others, are also known as *Karnapatrabhanga*. Woman in India never went around without earrings. On weddings and other festive days, the jewellery was so elaborate that earlobes had to be supported with chains tied up to different parts of the head.

✤ BHUSANA-YOJANA ✤

This is the art of making gold jewellery. Ornaments were considered to be of two varieties: the first included those strung on a thread: garlands of jewels, gems, pearls or other valuable stones. From the earliest times, the stringing together of flowers was an art. Garlands were offered in temples and were an important part of the evening-dress of both men and women. Even today garlands are exchanged during a wedding ceremony.

An honoured guest is welcomed with a garland. The other category included jewellery made of metals like gold and silver that were melted, then mixed with other materials to add colour and resilience and then be cast into different shapes. Ornaments like bangles, armlets, earrings, necklaces, waist belts were made by this process.

♣ SEKHARAKAPIDA-YOJANA ♣

This is a very specialized art of making ornaments using only flowers. *Sekharaka* denotes a type of flower ornament that is placed at the back of the head, that is on the *sikhasthana* and is then made to hang and encircle the neck like a *jhumka* (dangling earring). Besides this rather elaborate and intricately strung ornament, the hair was plaited with flowers from the top of the head right to the tip, intricate designs made to look as though they were made of gold and silver, depicting the sun and moon were worn on the top of the head. Elaborate bracelets, bangles,

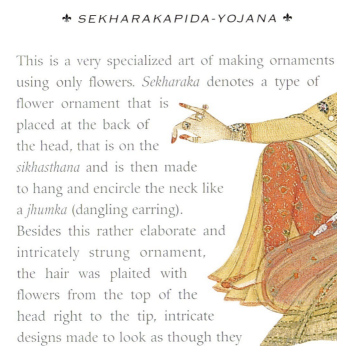

Women also embellished themselves with jewellery and flowers to please their lovers.

bajubands (armlets), waist bands were woven from fresh jasmine emphasizing the beauty of the thin waist besides adding fragrance.

♣ VISESAKACHHEDYA ♣

This is the art of painting the forehead with the mark; the word *visesaka* itself means the *tilak* on the forehead. The forehead was painted often with sandalwood, turmeric, *kasturi* (musk), vermilion paste. The art of drawing intricate patterns on the forehead has retained its fascination to the present day. Apart from the forehead other body parts like the chin, neck, palm, breasts were also painted. *Alta* (red colour) was applied on the hands and feet as was *mehendi* (henna), a tradition that has survived till today. Henna was applied on the hands especially of brides as the red colour imparted was considered to be auspicious because of its emotional, sexual and fertility-related qualities.

♣ GANDHA-YUKTI ♣

The use of perfumes is extremely ancient in India extolled even in the scriptures. Details of the manufacturing processes of perfumes appear in detail in a very well-known text: *Vrihatsamhita* by Varahamihira. Cosmetics, perfumes, deodorants, perfumed

Facing page: The body was considered to be a sacred temple, that had to be bathed in special oils and condiments.

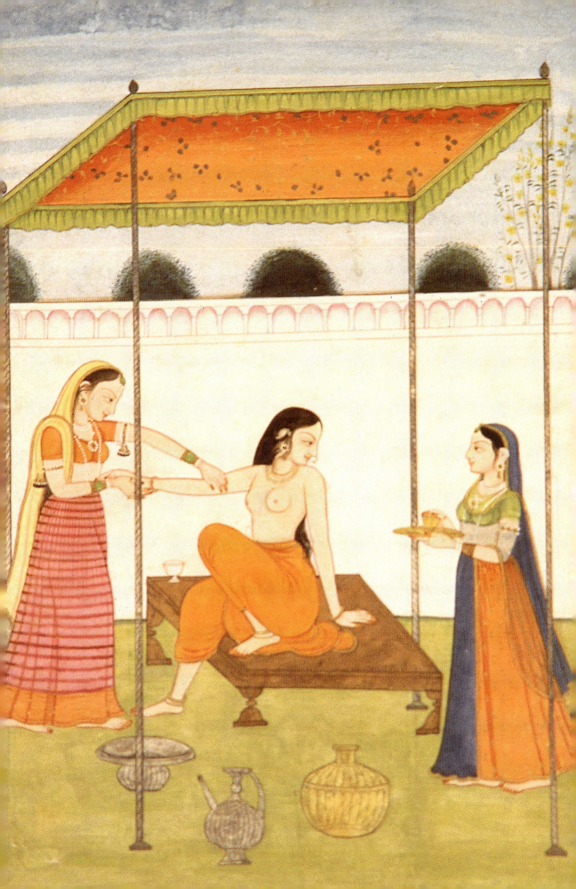

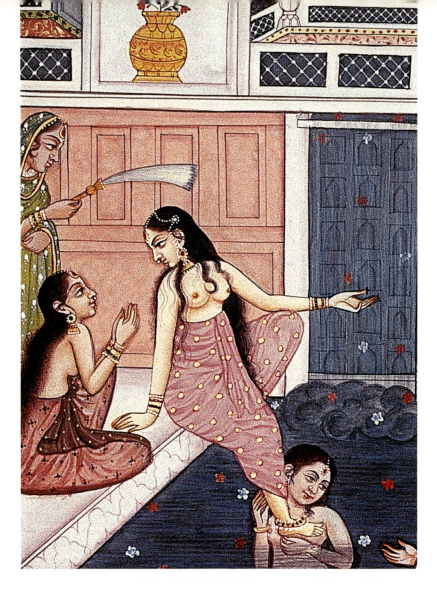

hair-oil, body creams, room fresheners, *agarbattis* and *dhoop* (incense) were made and used in copious quantities. It has been said that there were almost one lakh seventy-four thousand seven hundred and twenty methods for manufacturing perfumes. Rose water, sandalwood paste, musk, floral extracts like jasmine, rose, *champa* (frangipani), were all mixed and used imaginatively resulting in a bewildering array of fragrances.

A bath was an elaborate affair amidst an array of flowers and perfumes.

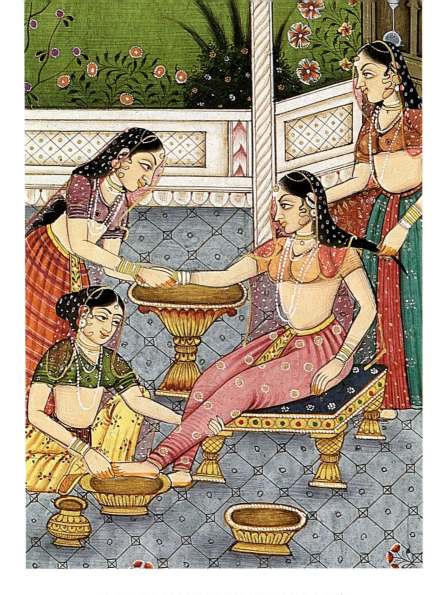

❖ DASSANAVASANANGARAGA ❖

Besides external ornamentation, the *Kama Sutra* also stresses the need for personal hygiene. Although this dwells on decorating the teeth, there was an equal emphasis on keeping them clean and sweet smelling at all times. The art itself was centered on painting the teeth, usually in gold or silver colours. Panini, the

---

Personal hygiene is of utmost importance in the act of love.

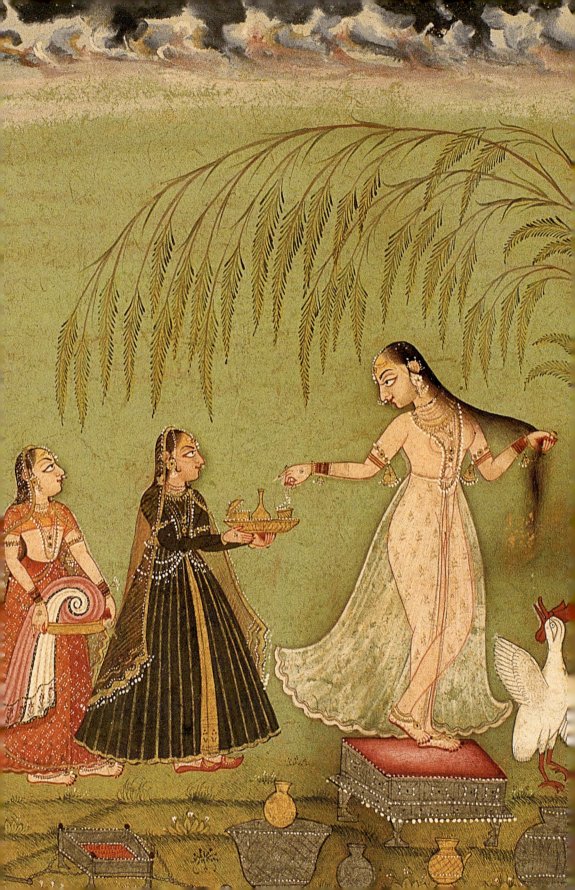

grammarian, makes a distinction between *dantalekhak* who is a painter of teeth and *nakhalekhak* a painter of nails. There are divisions within this art, all of which center around the use of colour, painting, dyeing and using colour on the face.

One such subdivision was known as *Vasanaraga* or the art of dyeing clothes, making coloured borders and printing floral impressions as well as embroidery work.

Another subdivision, *Angaraga*, was the use of colour for toiletry and make-up. Before the advent of designer creams, cosmetics were derived from natural sources—lac mixed with castor oil was used to paint lips, a fine powder called *lodhra-renu* was used on the face, lamp black used as kohl to outline the eyes, a mixture of gram powder, sandalwood powder and turmeric was used all over the body for cleansing. Some books talk about the technique of using a light alaktaka colour on the lip and then rubbing it with *sikthaka gutika* or candle wax balls, which would heighten the colour and make the lips shine.

Oils like almond, coconut, til oil were used all over the body and on the hair to keep it black, shiny and long. Other butter-based creams were used all over the body to keep the skin soft and supple. The purpose of *Angaraga* is not merely indulgence. Ancient Ayurvedic texts point out that if limbs and other parts of the body were properly rubbed down and cleansed, the body remained healthy and diseases were kept at bay.

Facing page: Women often wore their hair in very elaborate styles with flowers tucked in.

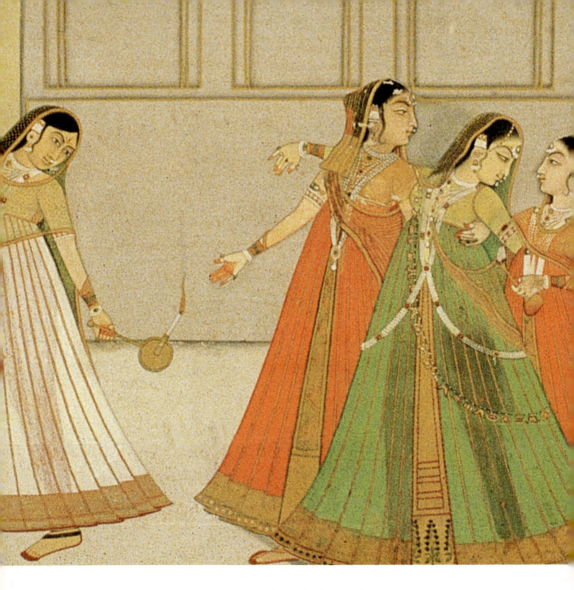

✣ VASTRAGOPANA ✣

This relates to the important art of couture, wearing clothes well, developing a style, and improvising. The text looks at how to wear clothes properly so that they do not slip off, how to improvise when new clothes are not available so that one always looks well dressed, and to wear even an ill fitting dress as a fitting one.

A good-looking woman stands out in society if she is also tastefully dressed.

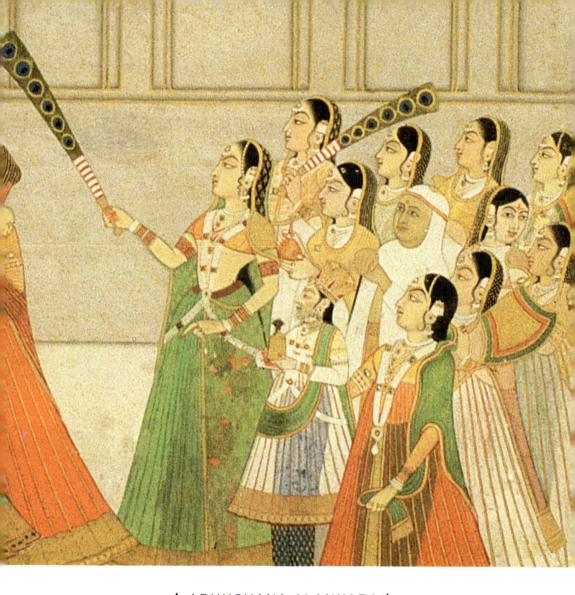

♣ ABHUSHANA ALANKARA ♣

The meaning of *bhushana* is to adorn and *abhushan* means ornaments meant to adorn. A good physique was always enhanced by wearing *abhushan* or ornaments. According to ancient texts there were scientific reasons for wearing ornaments: they affected the physical and mental well-being of a person. Silver was believed to be a cold metal and used to calm down an angry or agitated mind, whereas gold was considered to be hot, energizing a person besides ensuring ceremonial purity. It was believed that the use of these metals reduced the risk of cancer, and balanced blood circulation. Indians continue to revel in wearing jewellery: earrings, finger rings in all five fingers, toe rings, anklets, bangles, hair ornaments, pendants worn on the parting of the hair, waist bands, forearm bands, nose-rings all made out of pearls, precious gems, gold and silver. Indians studied gems and their effects on various ailments and temperaments. Astrologers too advised the use of gems to ward off the effects of planetary disturbances.

♣ KESHA SAMSKARA ♣

This focuses on the art of hairdressing. Long hair on women was seen as an *abhushan* or ornament enhancing the beauty of a woman. Elaborate hairstyles seen in the frescoes of Ajanta and Ellora and the sculptures of Belur and Halebid, were devised to enhance a woman's beauty. Elaborate ornaments were used to keep the hair in place and add to their allure.

Facing page: Long hair on a woman always adds to her beauty.

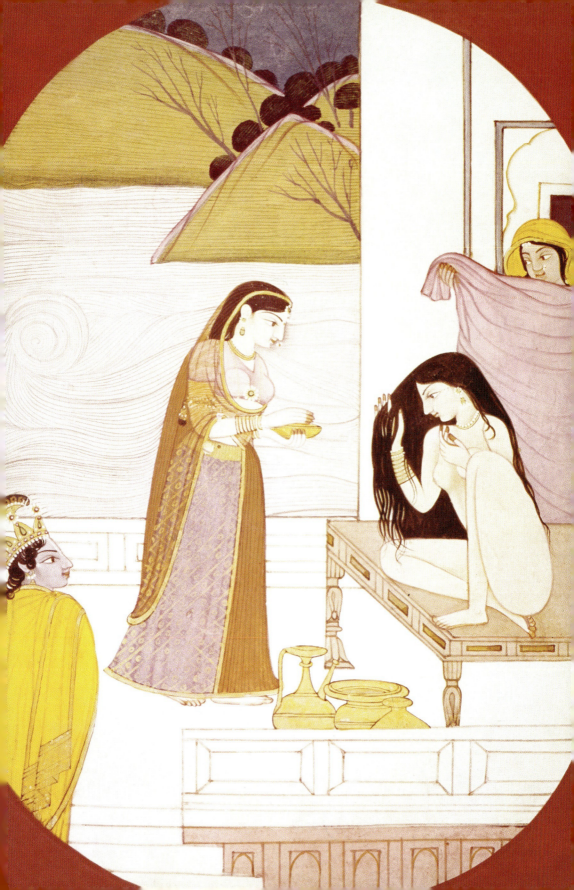

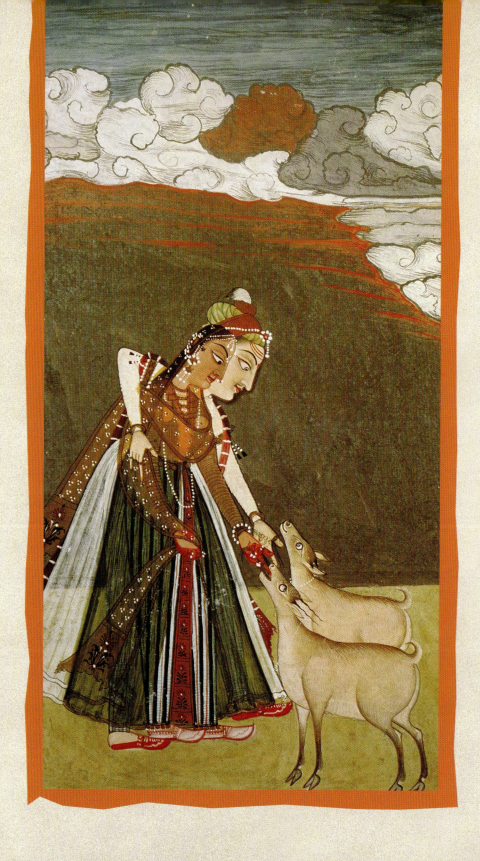

The Man and the Woman

Vatsyayana classifies men into three classes according to the size of their *lingam* or phallus: the hare man, the bull man, and the horseman.

He also classifies women according to the depth of their *yoni* or vagina: a female deer, a mare, or a female elephant.

There are thus three equal unions between persons of corresponding dimensions, and there are six unequal unions, when the dimensions do not correspond, or nine in all.

The equal unions are hare/deer; bull/mare; horse/elephant.

The unequal unions are hare/mare; hare/elephant; bull/deer; bull/elephant; horse/deer; horse/mare.

In these unequal unions, when the male exceeds the female in point of size, his union with a woman who is immediately next to him in size is called high union and is of two kinds; while his union with the woman most remote from him in

---

Facing page: In the union between a man and a woman, their physical attributes play a determining role.

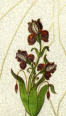

size is called the highest union, and is of one kind only. On the other hand, when the female exceeds the male in point of size, her union with a man immediately next to her in size is called low union, and is of two kinds; while her union with a man most remote from her in size is called the lowest union, and is of one kind only.

In other words, the horse and mare, the bull and deer, form the high union, while the horse and deer form the highest union. On the female side, the elephant and bull, the mare and hare, form low unions, while the elephant and the hare make the lowest union.

There are then, nine kinds of union according to dimensions. Amongst all these, equal unions are the best, those of a superlative degree, *i.e.*, the highest and the lowest are the worst, and the rest are middling, and with them the high are better than the low.

There are also nine kinds of union according to the force of passion or carnal desire. The three equal unions are when both partners have small, middling or intense passion. The unequal unions are small/middling; small/intense; middling/small; middling/intense; intense/small and intense/middling.

A man is called a man of small passion whose desire at the

time of sexual union is not great, whose semen is scanty, and who cannot bear the warm embraces of the female.

Those with a different temperament are called men of middling passion, while those of intense passion are full of desire. Similarly, women can be classified into three varying degrees of feelings as specified above.

And lastly, there are three kinds of men and women: the short-timed, the moderate-timed and the long-timed. When these diverse men and women meet, we have nine kinds of union.

But on this last point there is a difference of opinion about the female, which should to be clarified. Some say, 'Females do not emit as males do. The males simply remove their desire, while the females, from their consciousness of desire, feel a certain kind of pleasure, which gives them satisfaction, but it is impossible for them to tell you what kind of pleasure they feel. The fact from which this becomes evident is, that males, when engaged in coition, cease of themselves after emission, and are satisfied, but it is not so with females.

Others differ on the grounds that if a male is long-timed,

Following pages 86-87: Women's desires are not to be taken lightly, advises Vatsyayana.

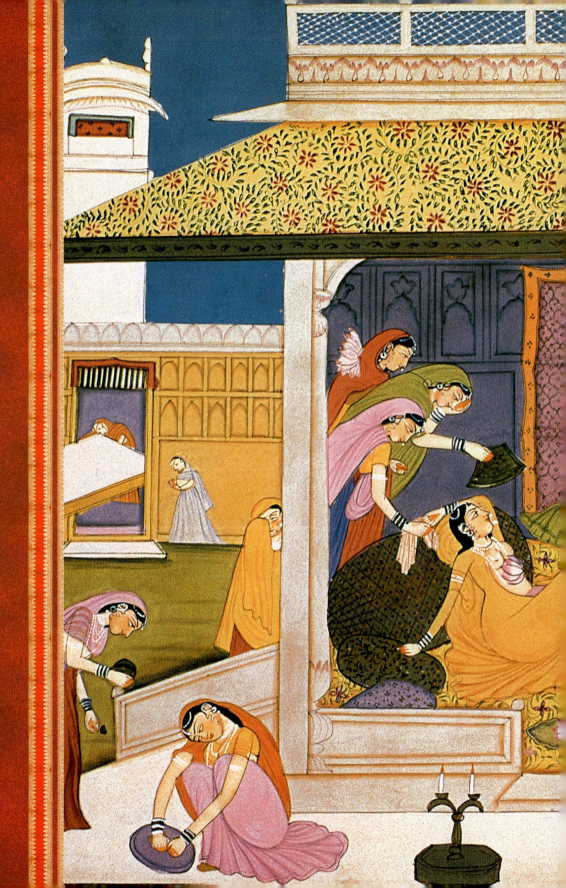

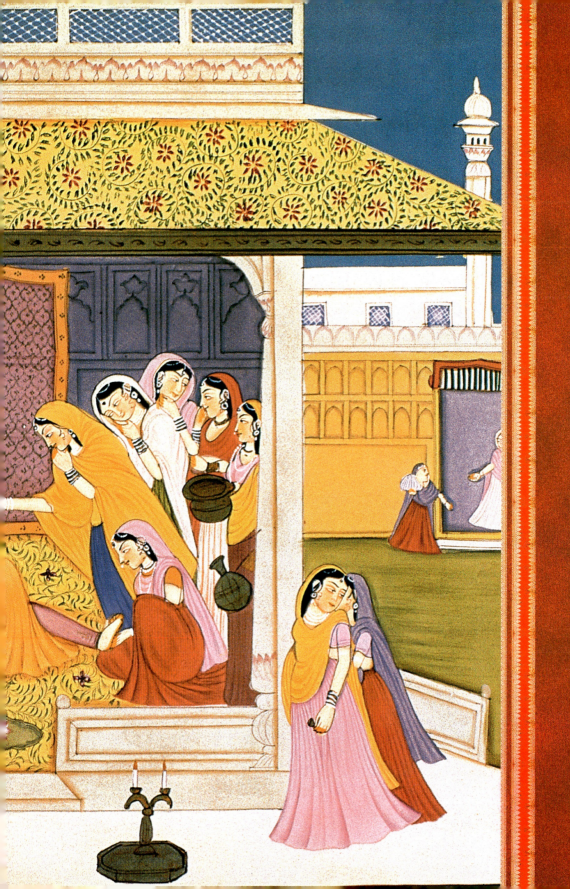

the female loves him the more, but if he is short-timed, she is dissatisfied with him. And this circumstance, some would say, would prove that the female emits also.

But this opinion does not hold well, for if it takes a long time to allay a woman's desire, and during this time she is enjoying great pleasure, it is quite natural then that she should wish for its continuation. And on this subject there is a verse as follows:

By union with men the lust, desire, or passion of women is satisfied, and the pleasure derived from the consciousness of it is called their satisfaction.

Some believe that the semen of women continues to fall from the beginning of the sexual union to its end, and it is right that it should be so, for if they had no semen there would be no embryo.
 To this there is an objection:

In the beginning of coition the passion of the woman is middling, and she cannot bear the vigorous thrust of her lover, but by degrees her passion increases until she ceases to think about her body, and then finally she wishes to stop from further coition.

Facing page: For a harmonious relationship, a man needs to satisfy the desires of the woman he loves.

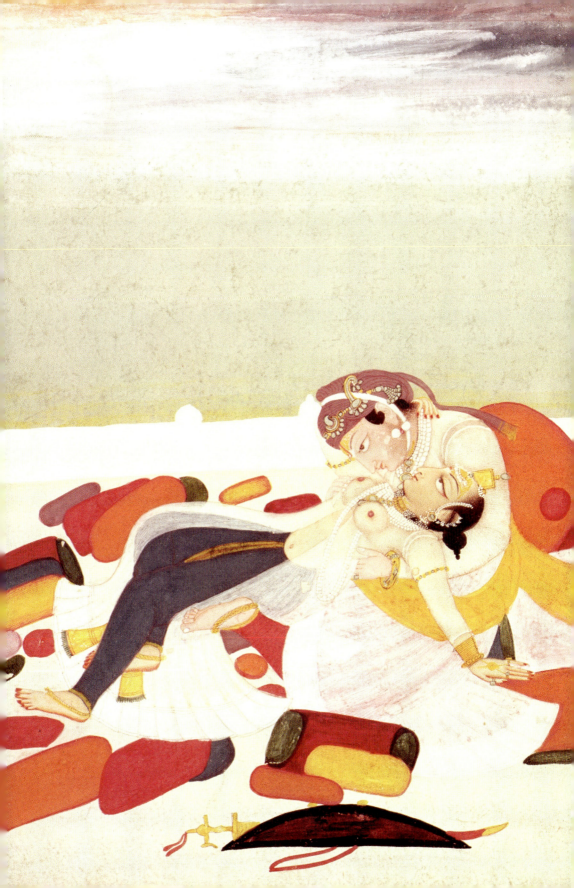

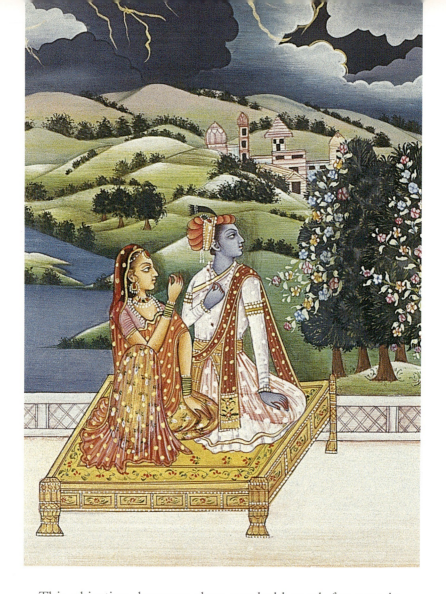

This objection, however, does not hold good, for even in ordinary things that revolve with great force, such as a potter's wheel, or a top, we find that the motion at first is slow, but by degrees it becomes very rapid. In the same way the passion of the woman having gradually increased she has a desire to discontinue coition, when all the semen has fallen away. And there is a verse with regard to this as follows:

The act of love must at all times be a mutually satisfying experience.

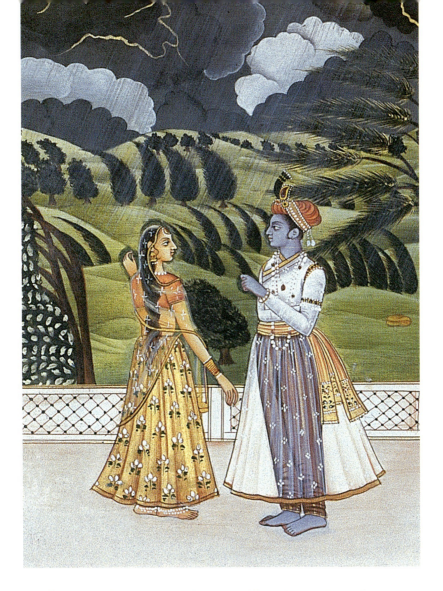

The fall of the semen of the man takes place only at the end of coition, while the semen of the woman falls continually, and after the semen of both has all fallen away then they wish for the discontinuance of coition.

In the final analysis, Vatsyayana is of the firm belief and opinion that the semen of the female falls in a manner rather similar to the way it does for the male.

The ultimate moment in love is no different from a spiritual union with God.

Now someone may ask here: if men and women are beings of the same kind, and are engaged in bringing about the same result, why should they have different works to do.

Vatsyayana says that this is so, because the ways of working as well as the consciousness of pleasure in men and women are different. The difference in the ways of working, by which men are the actors, and woman are the persons acted upon, is owing to the nature of the male and the female, otherwise the actor would be sometimes the person acted upon, and vice versa. And from this difference in the ways of working follows the difference in the consciousness of pleasure, for a man thinks, 'this woman is united with me,' and a woman thinks, 'I am united with this man.'

It may be said that if the ways of working in men and women are different, why should not there be a difference, even in the pleasure they feel, and which is the result of those ways.

But this objection is groundless, for the person acting and the person acted upon being of different kinds, there is a reason for the difference in their ways of working; but there is no reason for any difference in the pleasure they feel, because they both naturally derive pleasure from the act they perform.

Facing page: Pleasure holds the same import for a man and a woman.

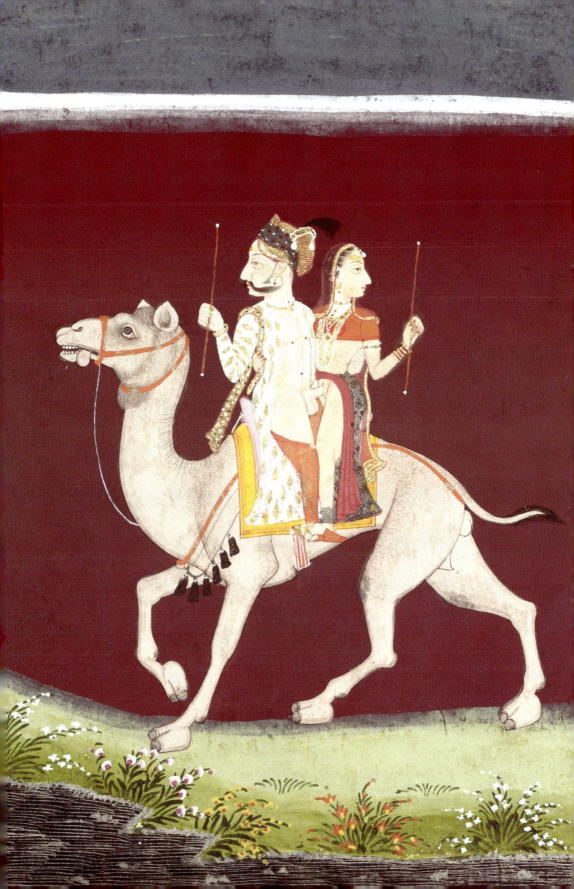

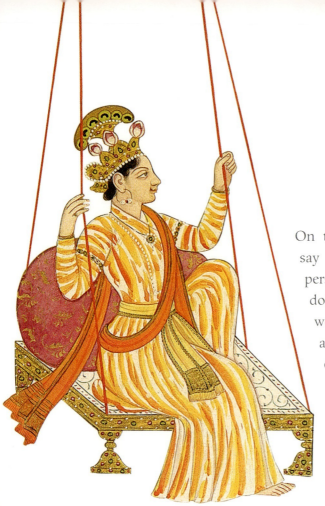

On this again some may say that when different persons are engaged in doing the same work, we find that they accomplish the same end or purpose; while, on the contrary, in the case of men and women we find that each of them accomplishes his or her own separately. This is inconsistent. But this is a mistake, for we find that sometimes two things are done at the same time, as for instance in the fighting of rams, both the rams receive the shock at the same time on their heads. Again, in throwing one wood apple against another, and also in a fight or struggle of wrestlers. If it be said that in these cases the things employed are of the same kind, it is answered that even in the case of men and women, the nature of the two persons is the same. And as the difference is of their conformation only, it follows that men experience the same kind of pleasure as women do.

A man should marry a woman who would be a willing accomplice in his game of seduction.

Men and women being of the same nature, feel the same kind of pleasure, and therefore a man should marry such a woman as will love him ever afterwards.

The pleasure of men and women being thus proved to be of the same kind, it follows that in regard to time, there are nine kinds of sexual intercourse, in the same way as there are nine kinds according to the force of passion.

There being thus nine kinds of union with regard to dimensions, force of passion, and time, respectively, by making combinations of them, innumerable kinds of union would be produced. Therefore in each particular kind of sexual union, men should use such means as they may think suitable for the occasion.

At the first time of sexual union the passion of the male is intense, and his time is short, but in subsequent unions on the same day the reverse of this is the case. With the female however it is the contrary, for at the first time her passion is weak, and then her time long, but on subsequent occasions on the same day, her passion is intense and her time short, until her passion is satisfied.

A woman plays a crucial role in prolonging the act of love.

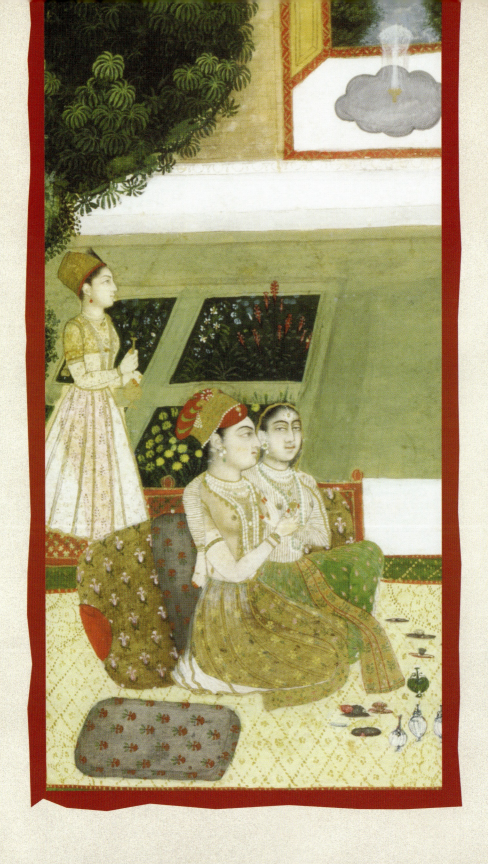

Love and Art

Love is a many-spendoured thing. It is a language of the heart and is so often portrayed through expressions of emotion. According to the *Kama Sutra* there are four kinds of love:

⚜ LOVE ACQUIRED BY CONTINUAL HABIT ⚜

Love resulting from the constant and continual performance of some act is called love acquired by constant practice and habit, as for instance the love of sexual intercourse, the love of hunting, the love of drinking, the love of gambling, etc.

⚜ LOVE RESULTING FROM IMAGINATION ⚜

Love which is felt for things to which we are not habituated, and which proceeds entirely from ideas, is called love resulting from imagination, as for instance, that love which some men and women and eunuchs feel for the *auparishtaka* or mouth congress, and that which is felt by all for such things as embracing, kissing, etc.

Facing page: Love is the language of the heart expressed through emotions.

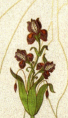

♣ LOVE RESULTING FROM BELIEF ♣

The love which is mutual on both sides, and proved to be true, when each looks upon the other as his or her very own, such is called love resulting from belief by the learned.

♣ LOVE RESULTING FROM PERCEPTION OF EXTERNAL OBJECTS ♣

The love resulting from the perception of external objects is quite evident and well known to the world, because the pleasure which it affords is superior to the pleasure of the other kinds of love, which exist for its sake.

♣ SIXTY-FOUR: A MAGICAL AND MYSTICAL NUMBER ♣

Traditionally, the arts are classified into *Nava Rasas* based on nine different emotions or moods: *srngara*/love, *hasya*/laughter, *karuna*/sadness, *raudra*/anger, *vira*/pride, *hayanaka*/fear, *bibhatsa*/disgust, *adbhut*/wonder and *shanta*/peace. Each raga was associated with a particular mood, and connected to a particular time of the day, year and season. The *Nava Rasas* set the foundation of the arts. The resulting sixty-four arts were conceived as channels of creative energy, considered direct emanations from the Goddess Saraswati, responsible in Indian mythology for learning besides being the muse for all the arts.

> The sixty-four arts are like the flames of an inner sun, blazing from the solar plexus, burning up negativity. These flames of creativity purify the psyche and bring about an inner transformation.

The number sixty-four in itself was also believed to be auspicious, being a legendary arithmetical figure in India, so that besides these branches of arts, there were sixty-four Mayas, sixty-four Yoginis, sixty-four Mudras, and so on.

Carefully cultivated, the pursuit of the arts was not left to chance, inspiration, individual taste or experience. *Chatushashtikala* or the sixty-four arts became an integral part of the curriculum and syllabus. Skill in at least some of the sixty-four arts established a woman's credentials, especially when she became of marriageable age, and was an indication of whether she would make a good wife and enthusiastic lover.

Some of the more important arts listed in the *Kama Sutra* are:

✤ MUSIC ✤

The first amongst the fine arts is considered to be music. The Chandogya Upanishad calls music the *Devajanavidya* or the knowledge of the Gods. The *Puranas*, also clearly show that a close relationship existed between religion and music as early as 1000 B.C.E and was considered to be a representation of divine beauty, a mediator between the spiritual and sensual life. A universal language often used to express beauty and joy,

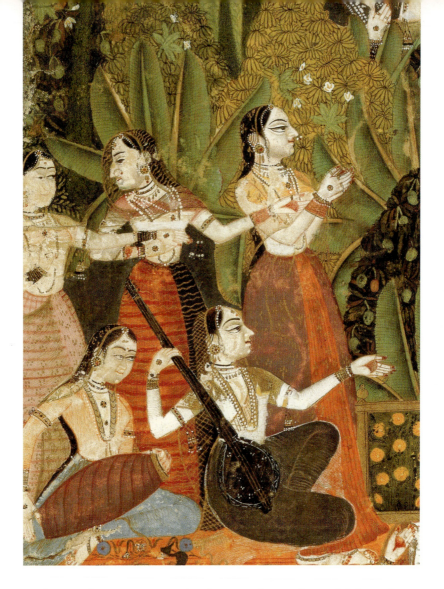

pathos and as prayer, music elevates the soul to a higher plane, making it possible to directly seek the divine. Learning and appreciating music naturally elevates a human being, making him more attuned to emotional nuances and thus more humane. The feminine aspect of a *raga* is known as the *ragini* and is synonymous with the *nayika* or the romantic heroine who is omnipresent in her myriad manifestations in Indian art and literature.

Music has always been closely associated with religion in the scriptures.

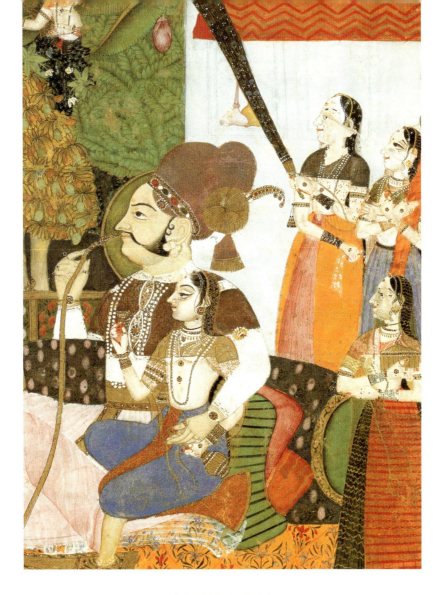

✤ DANCING ✤

Closely associated with music is dance that has been defined as a motion that arises from emotion. With its natural appetite for rhythm, the human body responds naturally to any vibrating sound. In India, the *Natya Shastras* as propounded by Bharata became the touchstone of this ancient art form. The relationship of the body, senses, mind, intellect and soul are all interlinked and

---

Music lends a variety of nuances to love, ranging from the erotic to the spiritual.

is regarded by Hindus as the abode of the divine. Therefore a beautiful body was seen as a temple of god and dance a medium for invoking the divine within.

♣ PAINTING AND SCULPTURE ♣

The *Navarasa bhava* found full expression in painting and sculpture. In the miniature paintings from Mewar or the Kangra Valley, idyllic nature scenes were created to convey a sense of joy and wonder, or a mood of unspoiled romance and eroticism. As was seen in the case of such themes as *nayika bheda* (differentiation of heroes and heroines) or the *ragamala* paintings, which took its cue from structural melodies, desire and devotion are combined in ingenious ways. The same sentiment also found expression in stone especially in temples like Khajuraho and Konarak where *Kama* merged with *Rasa* to form one of the most celebrated art forms that India has ever known.

♣ CULINARY SKILLS ♣

Amongst all the domestic arts, pride of place is occupied by the art of the palate. Housewives who won the hearts of their husbands through their stomachs are legion. In ancient India, a good cook held an honoured place in society; Draupadi was acknowledged to be a very good cook, as were Bhima and King Nala. Proficiency in cooking, imagination in serving a meal and catering to one's husband and his guests were and are still upheld as supreme virtues in India.

♣ CHEWING PAAN ♣

The word *tambula* occurs with regular frequency in most *Kama Shastra* texts being closely associated as a form of foreplay when the *nayak* and *nayika* first meet. The *Kama Sutra* says:

> Only after cleaning the teeth and having looked into the mirror and having eaten a *tambula* to render fragrance to the mouth, should a person start his day's work.

Tambula, which is basically a betel nut wrapped in a *paan* leaf is a Sanskrit word that derives its name from the word *tamra* (copper), indicating red colour. According to Sushruta, the patriarch of ancient Indian Ayurveda, *paan* keeps the mouth clean, strengthens the voice, tongue and teeth, guards against diseases besides being a digestive. Early Sanskrit texts mention the consumption of betel leaf among the eight enjoyments, some of the others being incenses, women, clothes, music, bed and food.

Dance reflects one of the highest levels of spiritual union between a couple.

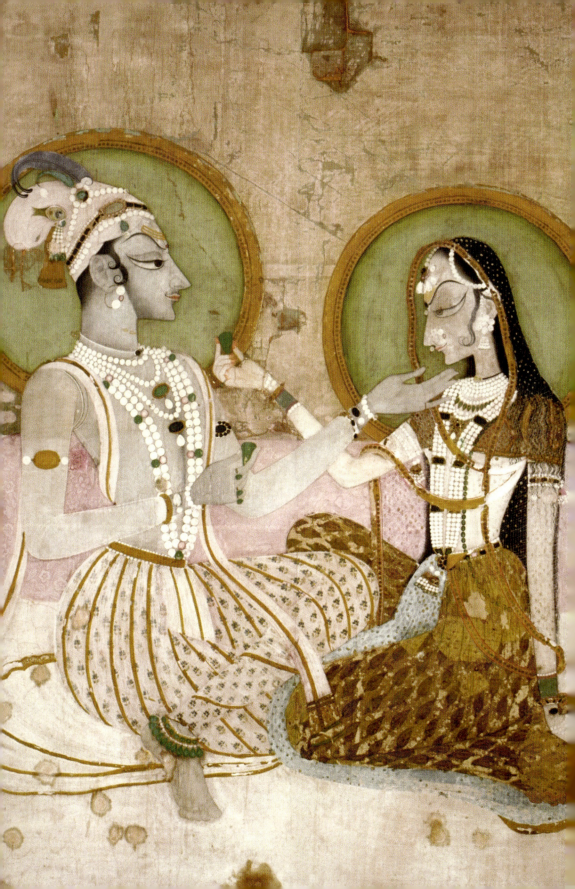

Offered in ritual and to the gods, Vatsyayana included the *tambula* as one of the *solah shringars* or 16 items of toiletries.

There are various opinions on why the part of the *Kama Shastra*, which treats sexual union, is called *Chatushashti*: sixty-four.

Some sages say that it is called so, because it contains sixty-four chapters. Other hold the opinion that the author of this part being a person named Panchala, and the person who recited the part of the Rig Veda called *Dashatapa*, which contains sixty-four verses, being also called Panchala, the name 'sixty-four' has been given to the part of the work in honour of the Rig Vedas.

Others say that this part contains eight subjects: the embrace, kissing, scratching with the nails or fingers, biting, lying down, making various sounds, playing the part of a man, and the *auparishtaka*, or mouth congress. Each of these subjects being of eight kinds, and eight multiplied by eight being sixty-four, this part is therefore named 'sixty-four'. But Vatsyayana affirms that as this part contains also the following subjects: striking, crying, the acts of a man during congress, the various kinds of congress, and other subjects, the name 'sixty-four' is given to it only accidentally.

Whatever may be the reason for this section being called sixty-four, the first subject to be considered here is the embrace.

Facing page: Lovers often offered each other paan *leaf as an initial step towards the final moment of pleasure.*

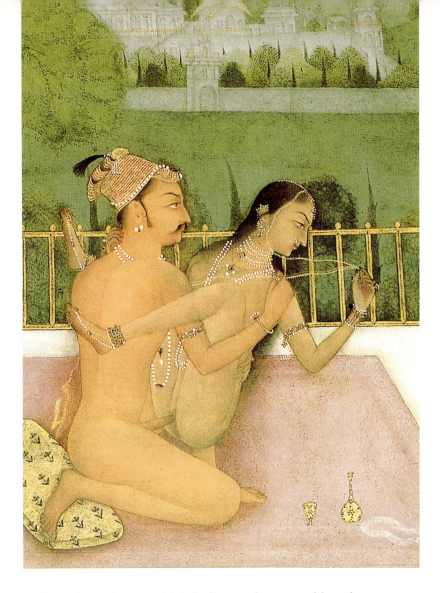

Now the embrace, which indicates the mutual love between a man and woman who have come together, is of four kinds:

♣ TOUCHING ♣

When he under some pretext or other goes in front of or alongside her and touches her body with his own, it is called the 'touching embrace'.

The Kama Sutra lists at least sixty-four different postures that a couple can try for variety.

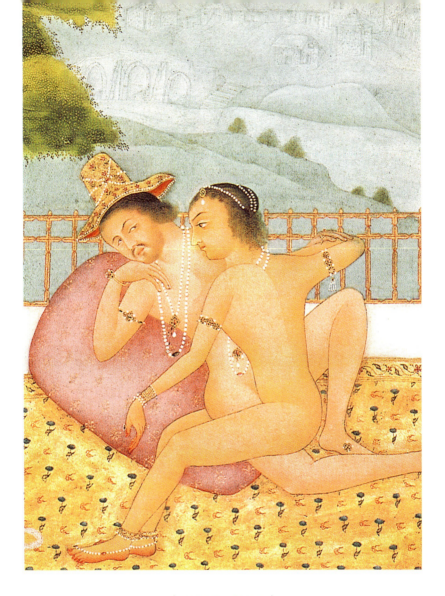

❖ PIERCING ❖

When she in a lonely place bends down, as if to pick up something, and pierces, as it were, the man sitting or standing, with her breasts, and he in return takes hold of them, it is called a 'piercing embrace'.

The above two kinds of embrace take place only

In the throes of love, kissing, biting, scratching are all permitted.

between persons who do not, as yet, speak freely with each other.

❧ RUBBING ❧

When two lovers are walking slowly together, either in the dark, or in a place of public resort, or in a lonely place, and rub their bodies against each other, it is called a 'rubbing embrace'.

❧ PRESSING ❧

When on the above occasion one of them presses the other's body forcibly against a wall or pillar, it is called a 'pressing embrace'.

These last two embraces are peculiar to those who know the intentions of each other.

At the time of meeting the following kinds of embrace are used:

❧ *JATAVESHTITAKA*, OR THE TWINING OF A CREEPER ❧

When she, clinging to him as a creeper twines round a tree, bends his head down to hers with the desire of kissing him and slightly makes the sound of *sut sut*, embraces him, and looks lovingly towards him, it is called an embrace like the 'twining of a creeper'.

♣ *VRIKSHADHIRUDHAKA*, OR CLIMBING A TREE ♣

When she, having placed one of her feet on the foot of her lover, and the other on one of his thighs, passes one of her arms round his back, and the other on his shoulders, makes slightly the sounds of singing and cooing, and wishes, as it were, to climb up him in order to have a kiss, it is called an embrace like the 'climbing of a tree'. These two kinds of embrace take place whilst the lover is standing.

♣ *TILA-TANDULAKA*, OR THE MIXTURE OF SESAME SEED WITH RICE ♣

When lovers lie on a bed, and embrace each other so closely that the arms and thighs of the one are encircled by the arms and thighs of the other, and are, as it were, rubbing up against them, this is called an embrace like 'the mixture of sesame seed with rice'.

♣ *KSHIRANIRAKA*, OR MILK AND WATER EMBRACE ♣

When she and he are very much in love with each other and, not thinking of any pain or hurt, embrace each other as if they were

---

Following pages 110-111: Indian scriptures are lavish in their descriptions of Radha and Krishna's love.

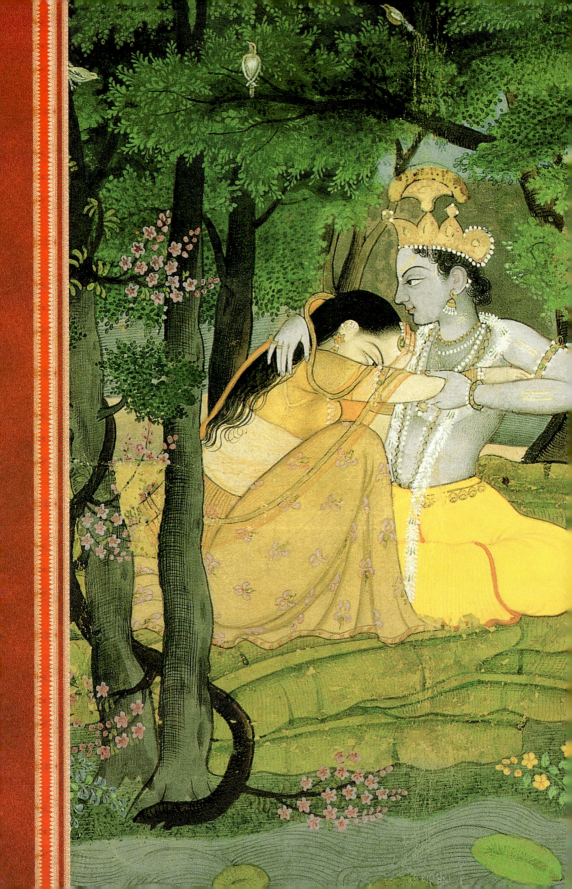

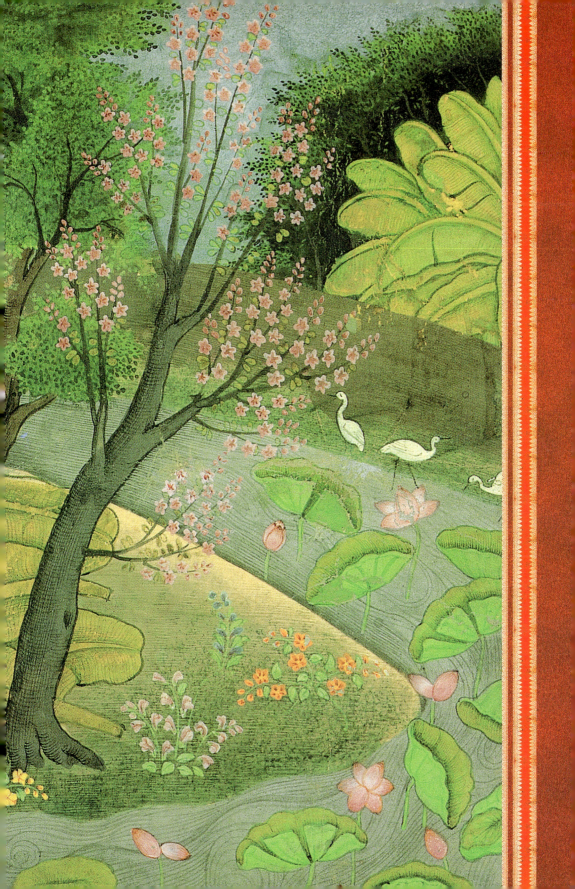

entering into each other's bodies either while the woman is sitting on the lap of him, or in front of him, or on a bed, then it is called an embrace like a 'mixture of milk and water'.

These two kinds of embrace take place at the time of sexual union. There are four ways of embracing simple members of the body, which are:

♣ THE EMBRACE OF THE THIGHS ♣

When one of two lovers presses forcibly one or both of the thighs of the other between his or her own, it is called the 'embrace of thighs'.

♣ THE EMBRACE OF THE *JAGHANA* ♣

When he presses the *jaghana* or middle part of her body against his own, and mounts upon her to practise, either scratching with the nail or finger, or biting, or striking, or kissing, her hair being loose and flowing, it is called the 'embrace of the *jaghana*'.

♣ THE EMBRACE OF THE BREASTS ♣

When he places his breast between the breasts of a woman and presses her with it, it is called the 'embrace of the breasts'.

Facing page: With practice, says Vatsyayana, one could easily perfect the postures described in the Kama Sutra.

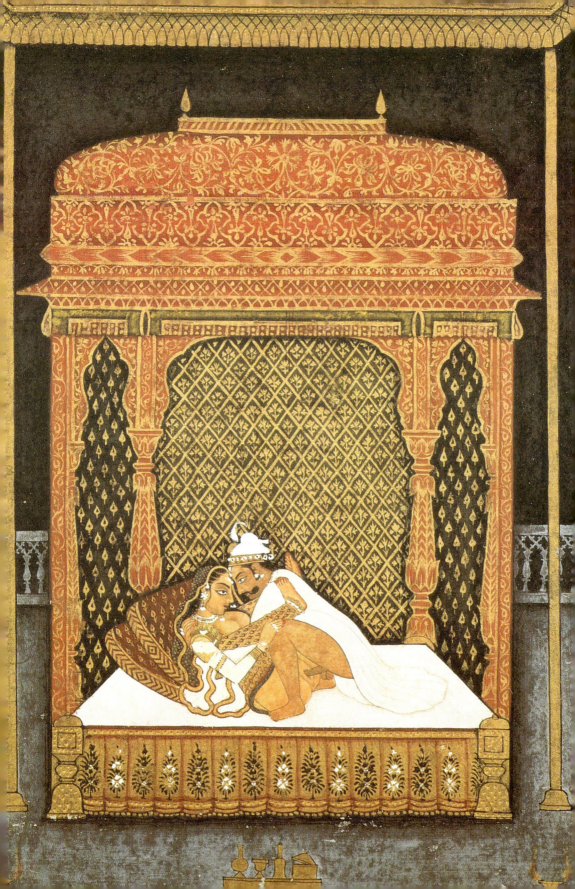

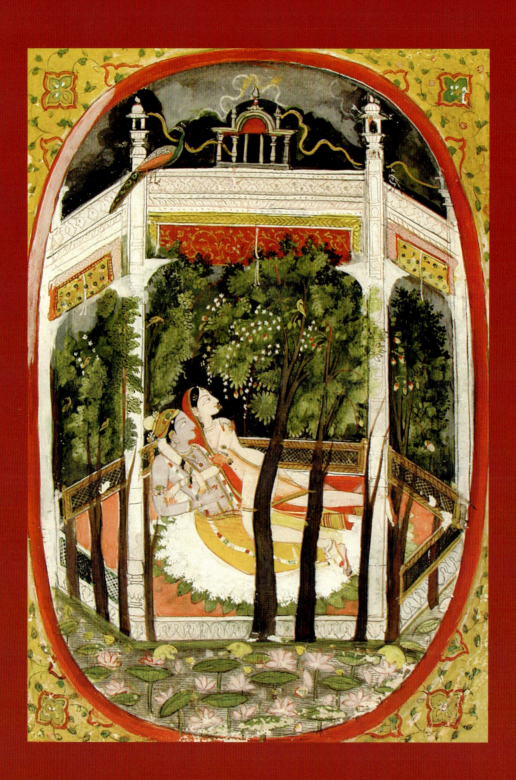

♣ THE EMBRACE OF THE FOREHEAD ♣

When either of the lovers touches the mouth, the eyes and the forehead of the other with his or her own, it is called the 'embrace of the forehead'.

> Some say that even shampooing is a kind of embrace, because there is a touching of bodies in it. But Vatsyayana thinks that shampooing is performed at a different time, and for a different purpose, and as it is also of a different character, it cannot be said to be included in the embrace.'

> The whole subject of embracing is of such a nature that men who ask questions about it, or who hear about it, or who talk about it, acquire thereby a desire for enjoyment. Even those embraces that are not mentioned in the Kama Shastra should be practised at the time of sexual enjoyment, if they are in any way conducive to the increase of love or passion. The rules of the Shastra apply so long as the passion of man is middling, but when the wheel of love is once set in motion, there is then no Shastra and no order.'

♣ KISSING ♣

'It is said by some that there is no fixed time or order

Facing page: Embracing each other gently and tenderly forms an important part of foreplay.

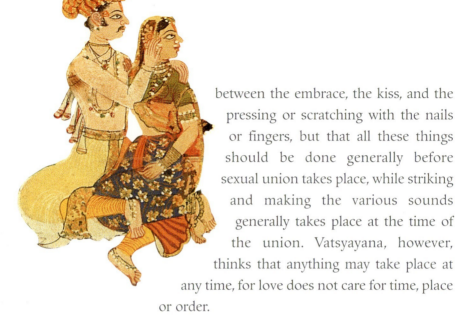

between the embrace, the kiss, and the pressing or scratching with the nails or fingers, but that all these things should be done generally before sexual union takes place, while striking and making the various sounds generally takes place at the time of the union. Vatsyayana, however, thinks that anything may take place at any time, for love does not care for time, place or order.

On the occasion of the first congress, kissing and the other things mentioned above should be done moderately, they should not be continued for a long time, and should be done alternately. On subsequent occasions however the reverse of all this may take place, and moderation will not be necessary, they may continue for a long time, and for the purpose of kindling love, they may all be done at the same time.

The following are the places for kissing: the forehead, the eyes, the cheeks, the throat, the bosom, the breasts, the lips, and the interior of the mouth. Moreover, the people of the Lat country kiss also the following places: the joints of the thighs, the arms, and the navel. But Vatsyayana thinks that

Lovers could embrace different parts of each other's body in order to stimulate desire.

though kissing is practised by these people in the above places on account of the intensity of their love, and the customs of their country, it is not fit to be practised by all.

In the case of a young girl there are three sorts of kisses:

♣ THE NOMINAL KISS ♣

When a girl only touches the mouth of her lover with her own, without doing anything else, it is called the 'nominal kiss'.

♣ THE THROBBING KISS ♣

When a girl setting aside her bashfulness a little, wishes to touch the lip that is pressed into her mouth, and with that object moves her lower lip, but not the upper one, it is called the 'throbbing kiss'.

♣ THE TOUCHING KISS ♣

When a girl touches her lover's lip with her tongue, and having shut her eyes, places her hands on those of her lover, it is called the *touching kiss.*'

Prolonging a kiss only serves to aggravate desire.

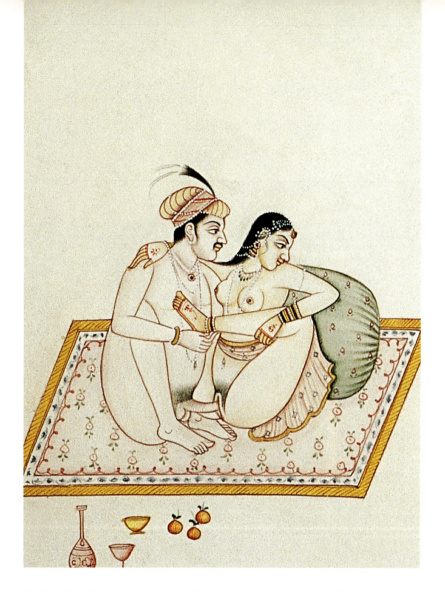

While the kisses described above are mentioned by Vatsyayana in the *Kama Sutra*, authors of various other treatises elaborated through the ages in India on sexuality and eroticism, either before the times of Vatsyayana, or even after him, have given detailed descriptions of various other different kinds of kisses. Amongst these are at least four more prominent forms of kisses that are not just suggested for young girls but for young and seasoned women as well. But there is no substitute for imagination and spontaneity.

Kissing different parts of the body removes sexual inhibitons between a couple.

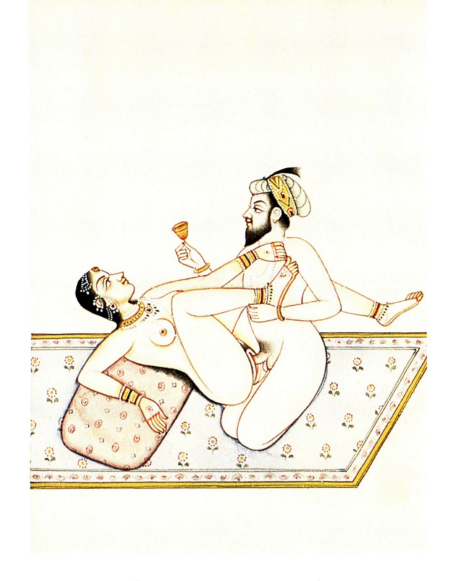

✣ THE STRAIGHT KISS ✣

When the lips of two lovers are brought into direct contact with each other, it is called a 'straight kiss'.

✣ THE BENT KISS ✣

When the heads of two lovers are bent towards each

There is nothing more desirable than a woman empowered.

other, and when so bent, kissing takes place, it is called a 'bent kiss'.

♣ THE TURNED KISS ♣

When one of them turns up the face of the other by holding the head and chin, and then kissing, it is called a 'turned kiss'.

♣ THE PRESSED KISS ♣

Lastly, when the lower lip is pressed with much force, it is called a 'pressed kiss'.

> There is also a fifth kind of kiss called the 'greatly pressed kiss' which is effected by taking hold of the lower lip between two fingers, and then after touching it with the tongue, pressing it with great force with the lip.
>
> As regards kissing, a wager may be laid as to which will get hold of the lips of the other first. If the woman loses, she should pretend to cry, should keep her lover off by shaking her hands, and turn away from him and dispute with him saying 'let another wager be laid'. If she loses this a second time, she should appear doubly distressed, and when her lover is off his guard or asleep, she should get hold of his lower lip, and hold it in her teeth, so that it should not slip away, and then she should laugh, make a loud noise, deride

him, dance about, and say whatever she likes in a joking way, moving her eyebrows, and rolling her eyes. Such are the wagers and quarrels as far as kissing is concerned, but the same may be applied with regard to the pressing or scratching with the nails and fingers, biting and striking. All these, however, are only peculiar to men and women of intense passion.

When he kisses the upper lip of a woman, while she in return kisses his lower lip, this is called the 'kiss of the upper lip'.

When one of them takes both the lips of the other between his or her own, it is called 'a clasping kiss'. She, however, only takes this kind of kiss from a man with no moustache. And on the occasion of this kiss, if one of them touches the teeth, the tongue, and the palate of the other, with his or her tongue, it is called the 'fighting of the tongue'. In the same way, the pressing of the teeth of the one against the mouth of the other is to be practised.

Kissing is of four kinds: moderate, contracted, pressed, and soft, according to the different parts of the body which are kissed, for different kinds of kisses are appropriate for different parts of the body.

When a woman looks at the face of her lover while he is

asleep, and kisses it to show her intention or desire, it is called a 'kiss that kindles love'.

When a woman kisses her lover while he is engaged in business, or while he is quarrelling with her, or while he is looking at something else, so that his mind may be turned away, it is called a 'kiss that turns away'.

When a lover coming home late at night, kisses his beloved who is asleep on her bed in order to show her his desire, it is called a 'kiss that awakens'. On such an occasion the woman may pretend to be asleep at the time of her lover's arrival, so that she may know his intention and obtain respect from him.

When a person kisses the reflection of the person she loves in a mirror, in water, or on a wall, it is called a 'kiss showing the intention'.

When a person kisses a child sitting on her lap, or a picture, or an image, or figure, in the presence of the person beloved by her, it is called a 'transferred kiss'. At night at a theatre, or in an assembly of caste men, he coming up to her kisses a finger, if she be standing, or a toe of her foot if she be sitting, or when she in shampooing her lover's body, places her face on his thigh (as if she was sleepy) so as to inflame his passion, and kisses his thigh or great toe, it is called a 'demonstrative kiss'.

Whatever things may be done by one of the lovers to the other, if the woman kisses him, he should kiss her in return, if she strikes him he should also strike her in return

♣ PRESSING, MARKING, OR SCRATCHING WITH THE NAILS ♣

When love becomes intense, pressing with the nails or scratching the body with them is practised, and it is done on the following occasions: on the first visit; at the time of setting out on a journey; on the return from a journey; at the time when an angry lover is reconciled; and lastly when the woman is intoxicated.

But pressing with the nails is not a usual thing except with those who are intensely passionate. It is employed together with biting, by those to whom the practice is agreeable.

Lovers' quarrels may be sorted out with a simple kiss.

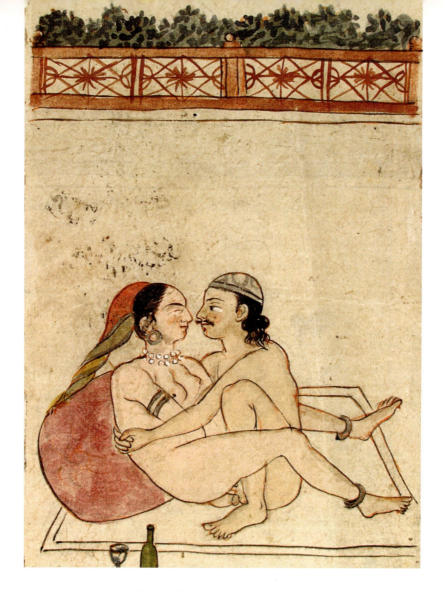

Pressing with the nails is of the eight following kinds, according to the forms of the marks which are produced.

The places that are to be pressed with the nails are as follows: the armpit, the throat, the breasts, the lips, the *jaghana*, or middle parts of the body, and the thighs. But Suvarnanabha is of the opinion that when the impetuosity of passion is excessive, then the places need not be considered.

Happiness and sexual equality belong to every human being.

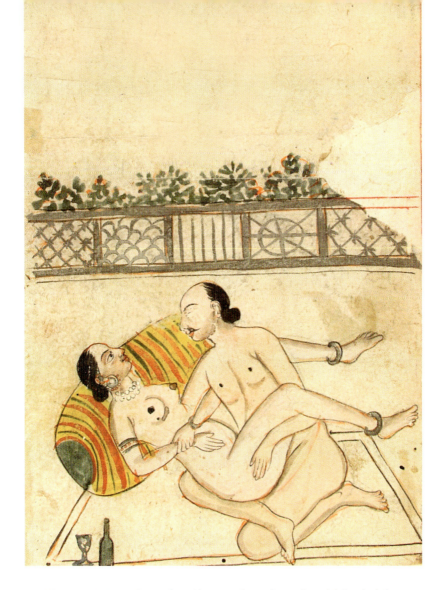

The qualities of good nails are that they should be bright, well set, clean, entire, convex, soft and glossy in appearance. Nails are of three kinds according to their size:

Small nails, which can be used in various ways, and are to be applied only with the object of giving pleasure.

Without eroticism, the physicality of sex is empty.

Middling nails, which contain the properties of both the above kinds.

Large nails, which give grace to the hands, and attract the heart from their appearance.

♣ SOUNDING ♣

When a person presses the chin, the breasts, the lower lip or the *jaghana* of another so softly that no scratch or mark is left, but only the hair on the body becomes erect from the touch of the nails, and the nails themselves make a sound, it is called a 'sounding or pressing with the nails'. This is used to shampoo, trouble or frighten a young girl.

♣ HALF MOON ♣

The curved mark with the nails, which is impressed on the neck and the breasts, is called the 'half moon'.

♣ A CIRCLE ♣

When the half moons are impressed opposite to each other, it is called a 'circle'. This mark with the nails is generally

Facing page: In order to give her great pleasure, a man must watch a woman's reactions carefully.

made on the navel, the small cavities about the buttocks, and on the joints of the thigh.

✣ A LINE ✣

A mark in the form of a small line, and which can be made on any part of the body, is called a 'line'.

✣ A TIGER'S NAIL OR CLAW ✣

This same line, when it is curved, and made on the breast, is called a 'tiger's nail'.

✣ A PEACOCK'S FOOT ✣

When a curved mark is made on the breast by means of the five nails, it is called a 'peacock's foot'. This mark is made with the object of being praised, for it requires a great deal of skill to make it properly.

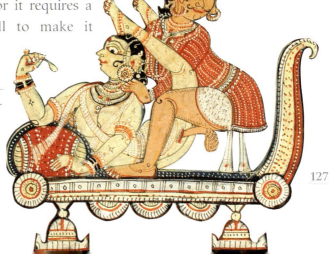

Following pages 128-129: Whatever be the setting, a man may need to instruct a woman on how to ignite the flames of passion.

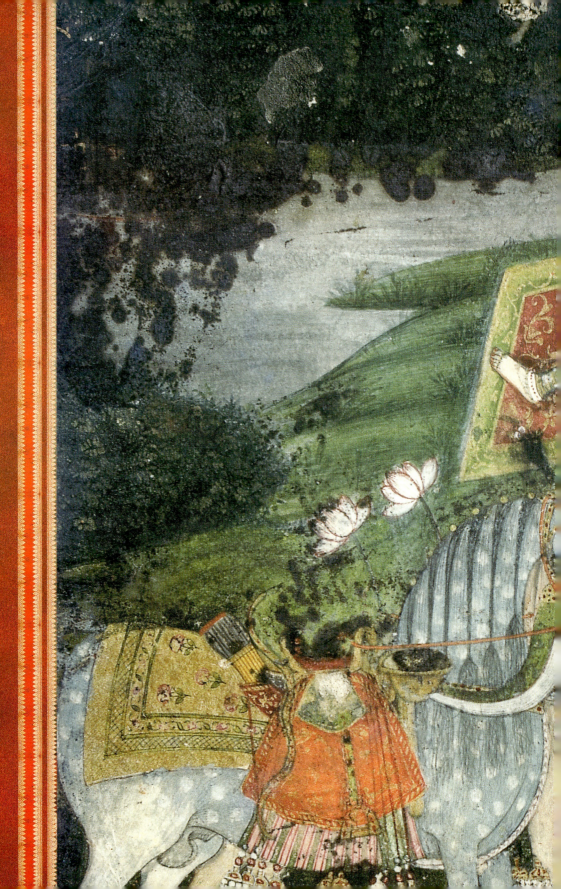

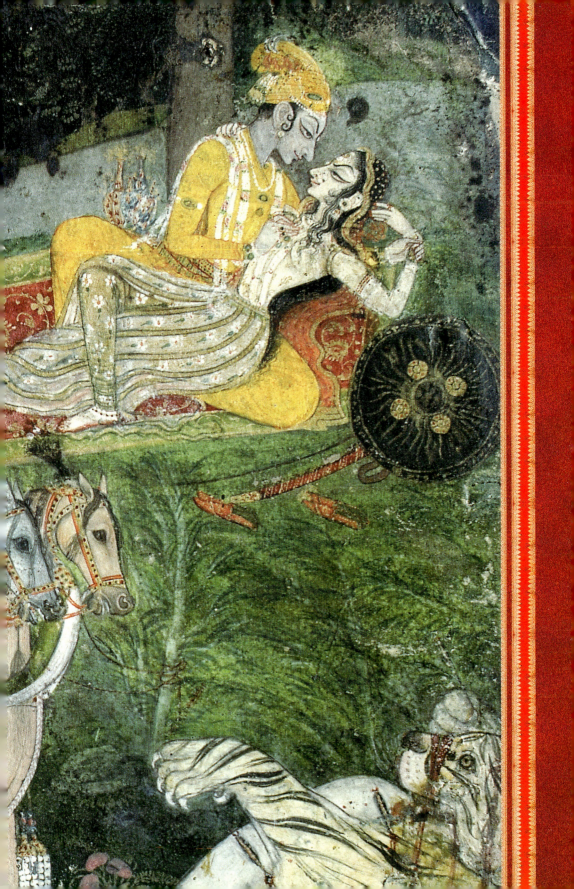

♣ THE JUMP OF A HARE ♣

When five marks with the nails are made close to one another near the nipple of the breast, it is called 'the jump of a hare'.

♣ THE LEAF OF A BLUE LOTUS ♣

A mark made on the breast or on the hips in the form of a leaf of the blue lotus, is called the 'leaf of a blue lotus'.

When a person is going on a long journey, and makes a mark on the thighs, or on the breast, it is called a 'token of remembrance'. On such an occasion three or four lines are impressed close to one another with the nails.

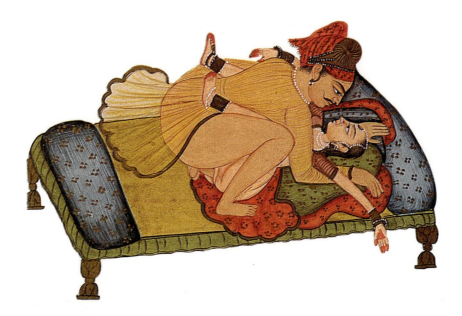

Here ends the marking with the nails. Marks of other kinds than the above may also be made with the nails, for the ancient authors say, that as there are innumerable degrees of skill among men (the practice of this art being known to all), so there are innumerable ways of making these marks. And as pressing or marking with the nails is dependent on love, no one can say with certainty how many different kinds of marks with the nails do actually exist.'

The reason for this is, as variety is necessary in love, so love is to be produced by means of variety. It is on this account that courtesans, who are well acquainted with the various ways and means, become so desirable, for if variety is sought in all the arts and amusements, such as archery and others, how much more should it be sought after in the present case.

The marks of the nails should not be made on married women, but particular kinds of marks may be made on their private parts for the remembrance and increase of love.

The love of a woman who sees the marks of nails on the intimate parts of her body, even though they are old and almost worn out, becomes again fresh and new. If there be no marks of nails to remind a person of the passages of love,

Facing page: To keep passion alive, reciprocity is essential.

then love is lessened in the same way as when no union takes place for a long time.

Even when a stranger sees at a distance a young woman with the marks of nails on her breast he is filled with love and respect for her.

A man, also, who carries the marks of nails and teeth on some parts of his body, influences the mind of a woman, even though it be ever so firm. In short, nothing tends to increase love so much as the effects of marking with the nails, and biting.

♣ BITING AND THE MEANS TO BE EMPLOYED ♣

All the places that can be kissed, are also the places that can be bitten, except the upper lip, the interior of the mouth, and the eyes.

The qualities of good teeth are as follows: They should be equal, possessed of a pleasing brightness, capable of being coloured, of proper proportions, unbroken, and with sharp ends.

Facing page: Variety and innovation in love ensure a long and satisfactory relationship.

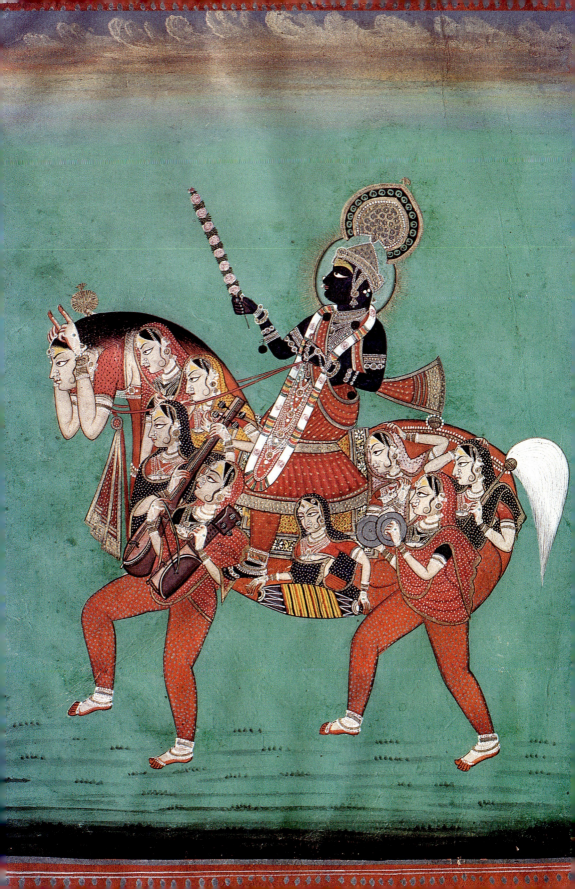

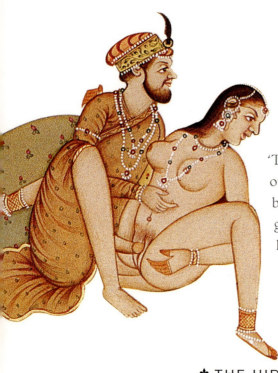

'The defects of teeth on the other hand are, that they are blunt, protruding from the gums, rough, soft, large and loosely set.'

The following are the different kinds of biting:

♣ THE HIDDEN BITE ♣

The biting which is shown only by the excessive redness of the skin that is bitten, is called the 'hidden bite'.

♣ THE SWOLLEN BITE ♣

When the skin is pressed down on both sides, it is called the 'swollen bite'.

♣ THE POINT ♣

When a small portion of the skin is bitten with two teeth only, it is called the 'point'.

Expanding sensual connections needs disciplining of the mind.

♣ THE LINE OF POINTS ♣

When such small portions of the skin are bitten with all the teeth, it is called the line of points'.

♣ THE CORAL AND THE JEWEL ♣

The biting which is done by bringing together the teeth and the lips, is called the 'coral and the jewel'. The lip is the coral, and the teeth the jewel.

♣ THE LINE OF JEWELS ♣

When the biting is done with all the teeth, it is called the line of jewels'.

♣ THE BROKEN CLOUD ♣

The biting which consists of unequal risings in a circle and which comes from the space between the teeth, is called the 'broken cloud'. This is impressed on the breasts.

♣ THE BITING OF THE BOAR ♣

The biting which consists of many broad rows of marks near to one another, and with red internals, is called the 'biting of a boar'. This is impressed on the breasts and the shoulders; and these two last modes of biting are peculiar to persons of intense passion.

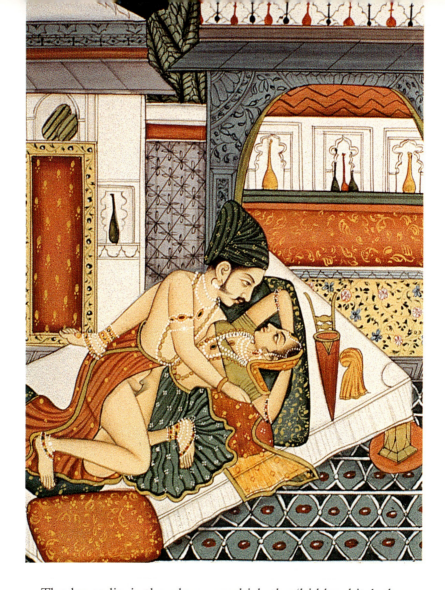

The lower lip is the place on which the 'hidden bite', the swollen bite, and the 'point' are made; again the 'swollen bite', and the 'coral and the jewel' bite are done on the cheek. Kissing, pressing with the nails, and biting are the ornaments of the left cheek, and when the word cheek is used, it is to be understood as the left cheek.

Both the 'line of points' and the 'line of jewels' are to be

Sexual candour and frankness between partners leads to the utlimate sexual pleasure for both.

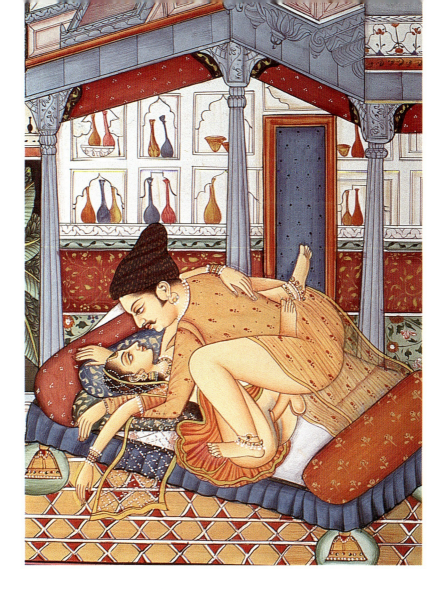

impressed on the throat, the armpit and the joints of the thighs; but the 'line of points' alone is to be impressed on the forehead and the thighs.

The nail markings, and the biting of the following things: a forehead or an ear ornament, a bunch of flowers, a betel leaf, or a *tamala* leaf, which are worn by, or belong to her that is beloved, are signs of the desire of enjoyment.

The act of love should be devoid of sexual guilt and any notion of sin.

Among the things mentioned above, (embracing, kissing, etc.,) those that increase passion should be done first, and those, which are only for amusement or variety, should be done afterwards.

When a man bites a woman forcibly, she should angrily do the same to him with double force. Thus a 'point' should be returned with a 'line of points', and a line of points' with a 'broken cloud', and if she be excessively chafed, she should at once begin a love quarrel with him. At such time she should take hold of her lover by the hair, and bend his head down, and kiss his lower lip, and then, being intoxicated with love, she should shut her eyes and bite him in various places. Even by day, and in a place of public resort, when her lover shows her any mark that she may have inflicted on his body, she should smile at the sight of it, and turning her face as if she were going to chide him, she should show him with an angry look the marks on her own body that have been made by him. Thus if he and she act according to each other's likes; their love for each other will not be lessened even in one hundred years.

Facing page: Feigning anger in passionate embrace only heightens the intensity of pleasure.

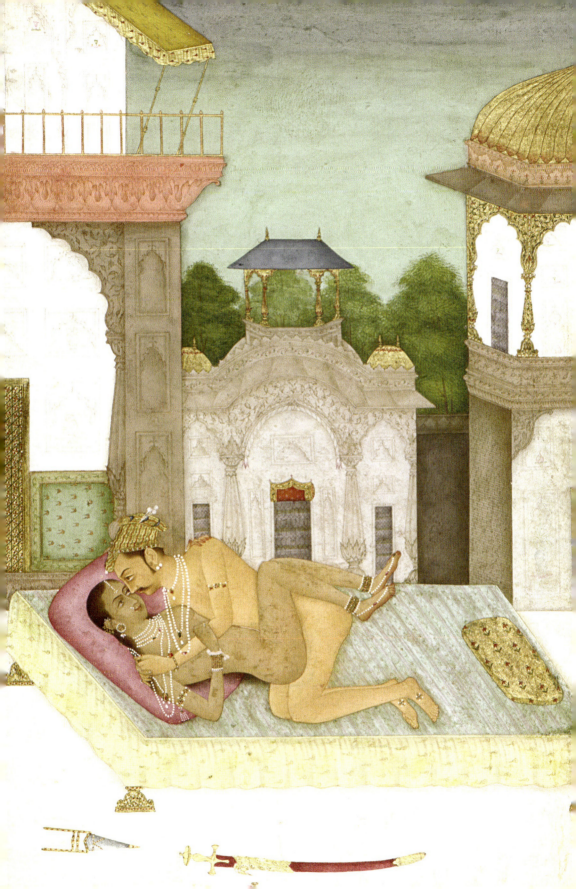

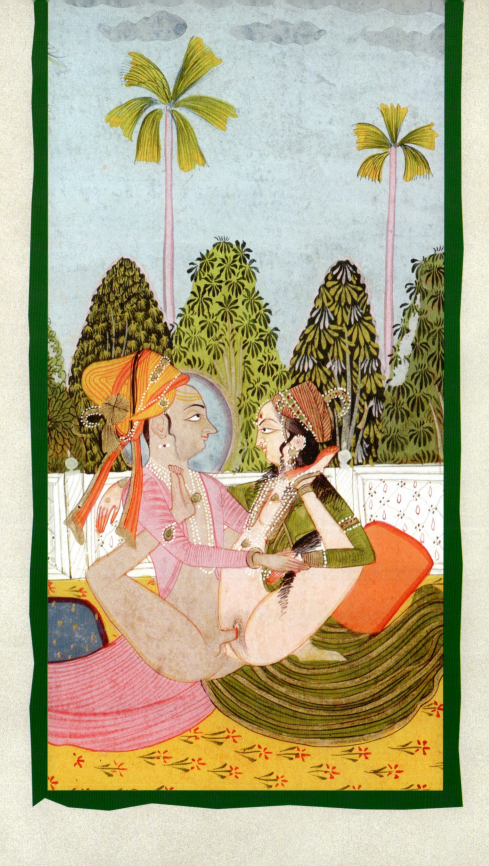

Play of Passion

Expanding sensual connections needs personal maturity, attentiveness and disciplining the mind as much as it requires disciplining the body. The solution, says Vatsyayana, lies in striking the right balance between all the human urges: physical, emotional, intellectual, social, sexual and spiritual. Compatibility is the key to true pleasure, so partners must suit each other in every respect: be it in temperament, the extent of passion, their physique, even the size of their genital organs. With a comprehensive understanding of inter-personal relationships, the *Kama Sutra* offers very urbane insights for satisfactory sex and ways to overcome tedium:

> The chief reason for the separation between husband and wife; the cause that drives the husband to the embraces of strange women and the wife to the arms of strange men is the want for varied pleasures and the monotony that follows possession. Monotony begets satiety and satiety (begets) distaste for congress and soon one or the other yields to temptation. It seldom happens that the two love each other

---

Facing page: Partners must suit each other in temperament and extent of passion.

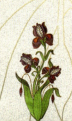

equally therefore the one is more easily seduced by passion than the other. The first consideration for a satisfactory sex life is that coition should be attempted only when both parties are inclined towards it; the second consideration is that intercourse should be preceded by such acts of love as would stimulate both partners equally. The third consideration is that the act should be undertaken in a posture, which would give maximum amount of pleasure and satisfaction. The posture adopted should be constantly varied to prevent monotony and preferences should be given to those postures where maximum mutual caresses are possible.

On the occasion of a 'high congress' the *Mrigi* or Doe-woman should lie down in such a way as to widen her *yoni*, while in a 'low congress' the *Hastini* or She-elephant woman who has a large vagina should lie down so as to contract hers. But in an 'equal congress' they should lie down in the natural position. What is said above concerning the *Mrigi* and the *Hastini* applies also to the *Vadawa* (Mare) woman. In a low congress' the woman should particularly make use of medicine, to cause her desires to be satisfied quickly.

The Deer woman has the following three ways of lying down.

♣ THE WIDELY OPENED POSITION ♣

When she lowers her head and raises her middle parts, it is called the 'widely opened position'. At such time the man should apply some lubricant, so as to make the entrance easy.

♣ THE YAWNING POSITION ♣

When she raises her thighs and keeps them wide apart and engages in congress, it is called the 'yawning position'.

♣ THE POSITION OF THE WIFE OF INDRA ♣

When she places her thighs with her legs doubled on them upon her sides, and thus engages in congress, it is called the position of Indrani, and this is learnt only by practice. The position is also useful in the case of the 'highest congress', together with the 'pressing position', the 'twining position', and the 'mare's position'.

When the legs of both the male and the female are stretched straight out

The ideal husband must submit to his wife and yet be the master of his destiny.

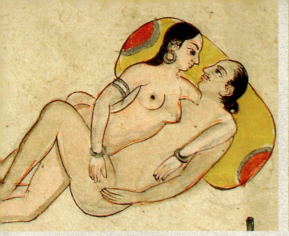 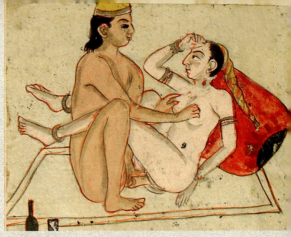

over each other, it is called the 'clasping position'. It is of two kinds, the side position and the supine position, according to the way in which they lie down. In the side position the male should invariably lie on his left side, and cause the woman to lie on her right side, and this rule is to be observed in lying down with all kinds of women.

When, after congress has begun in the clasping position, the woman presses her lover with her thighs, it is called the 'pressing position'.

When the woman places one of her thighs across the thigh of her lover, it is called the 'twining position'.

When the woman forcibly holds in her *yoni* the *lingam* after it is in, it is called the 'mare's position'. This is learnt by much practice only.'

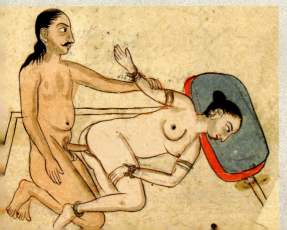 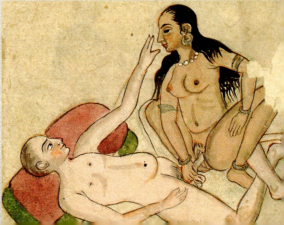

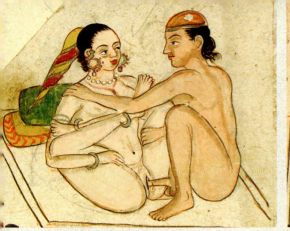 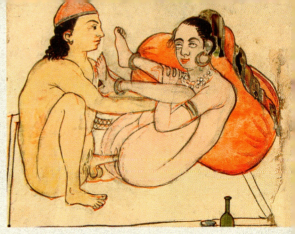

The above are the different ways of lying down. However, there are the following in addition:

When the female raises both of her thighs straight up, it is called the 'rising position'.

When she raises both of her legs, and places them on her lover's shoulders, it is called the 'yawning position'.

When the legs are contracted, and thus held by the lover before his bosom, it is called the 'pressed position'.

When only one of her legs is stretched out, it is called the 'half pressed position'.

When the woman places one of her legs on her lover's shoulder and stretches the other out, and then places the latter on his shoulder, and stretches out the other, and

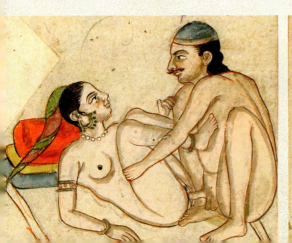 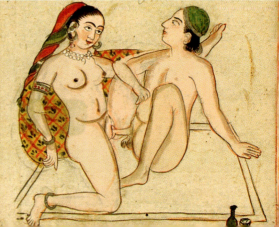

continues to do so alternately, it is called the 'splitting of a bamboo'.

When one of her legs is placed on the head, and the other is stretched out, it is called the 'fixing of a nail'. This is learnt by practice only.

When both the legs of the woman are contracted, and

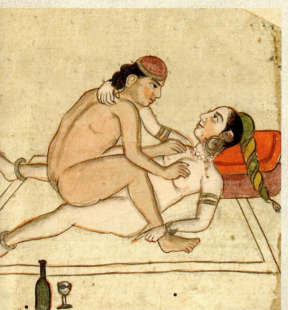
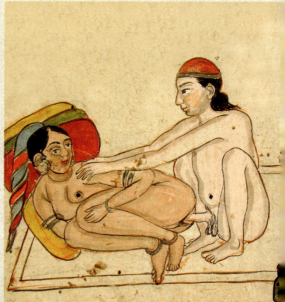

placed on her stomach, it is called the 'crab's position'.

When the thighs are raised and placed one upon the other, it is called the 'packed position'.

When the shanks are placed one upon the other, it is called the 'lotus-like position'.

When a man, during congress, turns round, and enjoys the woman without leaving her, while she embraces him round the back all the time, it is called the 'turning position', and is learnt only by practice.

Thus, says Suvarnanabha, these different ways of lying down, sitting, and standing should be practised in water, because it is easy to do therein. But Vatsyayana frowns upon this, because he

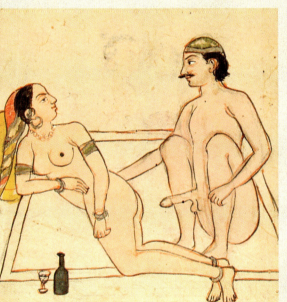
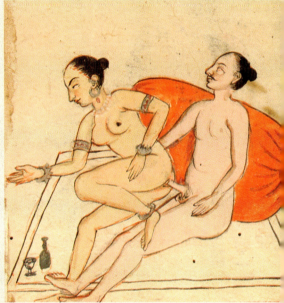

is of the opinion that congress in water is improper, because the religious law prohibits it.

When a man and a woman support themselves on each other's bodies, or on a wall, or pillar, and thus while standing engage in congress, it is called the 'supported congress'.

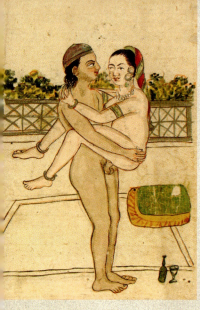

When a man supports himself against a wall, and the woman, sitting on his hands joined together and held underneath her, throws her arms round his neck, and putting her thighs alongside his waist, moves herself by her feet, which are touching the wall against which the man is leaning, it is called the 'suspended congress'.

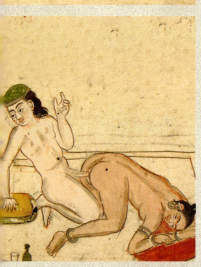

When a woman stands on her hands and feet like a quadruped and her lover mounts her like a bull, it is called the 'congress of a cow'. At this time everything that is ordinarily done on the bosom should be done on the back. In the same way can be carried on the congress of the dog, the congress of a goat, the congress of a deer, the forcible mounting of an ass, the congress of a cat, the jump of a tiger, the pressing of an elephant, the rubbing of a boar, and the mounting of a horse. And in all these acting like them should manifest the characteristics of these different animals.

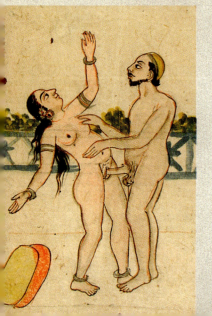

When a man enjoys two women at the same time, both of who love him equally, it is called the 'united congress'.

When a man enjoys many women

altogether, it is called the 'congress of a herd of cows'.

The following kinds of congress: sporting in water, or the congress of an elephant with many female elephants which is said to take place only in the water, the congress of a collection of goats, the congress of a collection of deer, take place in imitation of these animals.

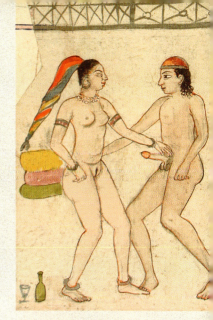

Many young men enjoy a woman that may be married to one of them, either one after the other, or at the same time. Thus one of them holds her, another enjoys her, a third uses her mouth, a fourth holds her middle part and in this way they go on enjoying her several parts alternately.

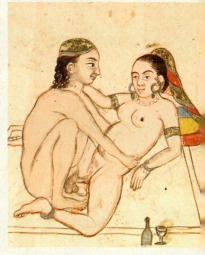

The same things can be done when several men are sitting in company with one courtesan, or when one courtesan is alone with many men. In the same way the women of the King's harem can do this when they chance upon a man by sheer accident.

The people in the some countries have also a congress in the anus that is called the 'lower congress'.

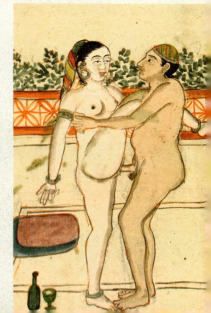

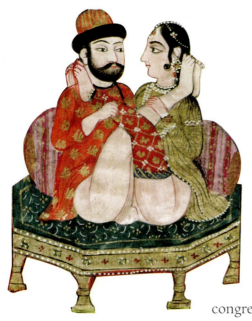

Thus ends the various kinds of congress. There are also two verses on the subject as follows:

An ingenious person should multiply the kinds of congress after the fashion of the different kinds of beasts and of birds. For these different kinds of congress, performed according to the usage of each country, and the liking of each individual, generate love, friendship, and respect in the hearts of women.

Sexual intercourse may be compared to a quarrel, on account of the contrarieties of love and its tendency to dispute. It is interesting, however, to note that there are no permanent disputes in love. The place of striking with passion is the body, and on the body the special places are:

♣ The shoulders
♣ The back
♣ The head
♣ The *jaghana* or middle part of the body
♣ The space between the breasts
♣ The sides

It is said that there is no fixed time for love.

Striking is of four kinds:

♣ Striking with the back of the hand
♣ Striking with the fist
♣ Striking with the fingers a little contracted
♣ Striking with the open palm of the hand

On account of its causing pain, striking gives rise to the hissing sound, which is of various kinds, and to the eight kinds of crying:

♣ The sound *hin*
♣ The sound *phut*
♣ The thundering sound
♣ The sound *phat*
♣ The cooing sound
♣ The sound *sut*
♣ The weeping sound
♣ The sound *plat*

Besides these, there are also words having a meaning, such as 'mother', and those that are expressive of prohibition, sufficiency, desire of liberation, pain or

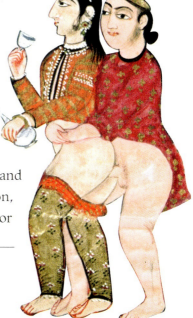

Couples are encouraged to try different postures in order to renew their love for each other.

praise, and to which may be added sounds like those of the dove, the cuckoo, the green pigeon, the parrot, the bee, the sparrow, the flamingo, the duck, and the quail, which are all occasionally made use of.

Blows with the fist should be given on the back of the woman, while she is sitting on the lap of the man, and she should give blows in return, abusing the man as if she were angry, and making the cooing and the weeping sounds. While the woman is engaged in congress the space between the breasts should be struck with the back of the hand slowly at first, and then proportionately to the increasing excitement, until the end.

At this time the sounds *hin* and others may be made, alternatively or optionally, according to habit. When the man, making the sound, *phat*, strikes the woman on the head, with the fingers of his hand a little contracted, it is called, *prasritaka*, which means striking with the fingers of the hand a little contracted. In this case the appropriate sounds are the cooing sound, the sound, *phat* and the sound, *phut* in the interior of the mouth, and at the end of congress the sighing and weeping sounds. The sound, *phat* is an imitation of the sound of a bamboo being split while the sound, *phut* is like the sound made by something falling

Facing page: The ancients suggest a series of sounds lovers are to make to enhance their lovemaking.

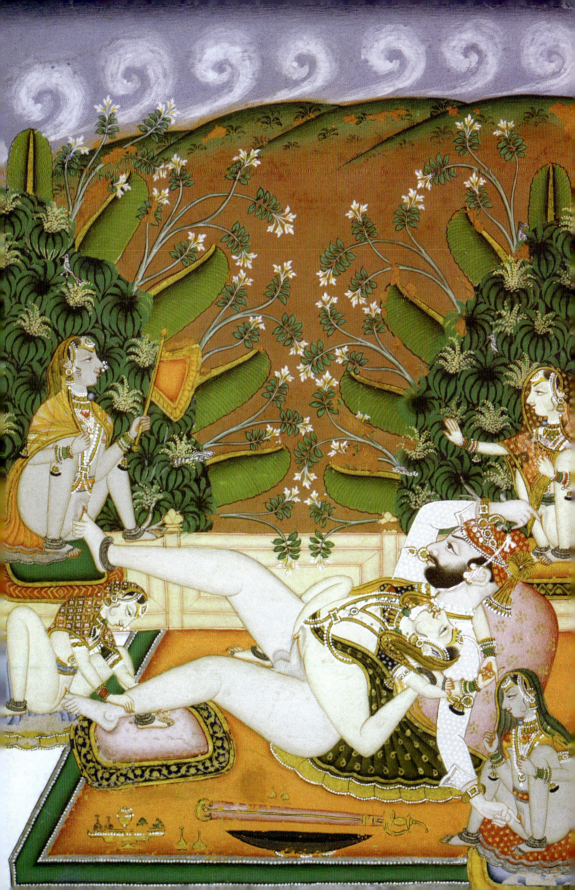

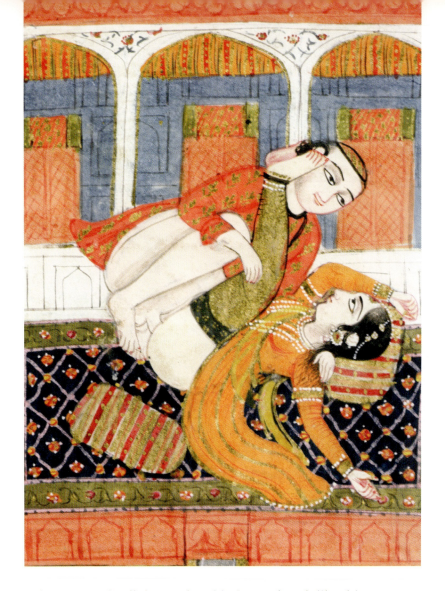

into water. At all times when kissing and such like things are begun, the woman should give a reply with a hissing sound. During the excitement when the woman is not accustomed to striking, she continually utters words expressive of prohibition, sufficiency or desire of liberation, as well as the words 'father,' 'mother' intermingled with the sighing, weeping and thundering sounds. Towards the conclusion of the congress, the breasts, the *jaghana*, and the sides of the

---

A seasoned woman would know how to give pleasure to her man.

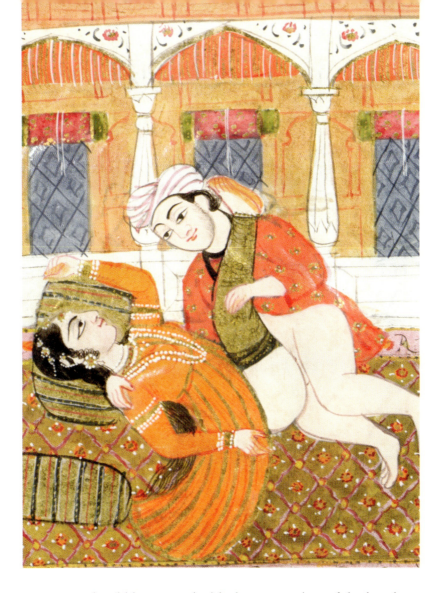

woman should be pressed with the open palms of the hand, with some force, until the end of it, and then sounds like those of the quail, or the goose should be made.

The characteristics of manhood are said to consist of roughness and impetuosity, while weakness, tenderness, sensibility, and an inclination to turn away from unpleasant things are the distinguishing marks of womanhood. The

A woman's reactions during lovemaking provide the right cue to her lover.

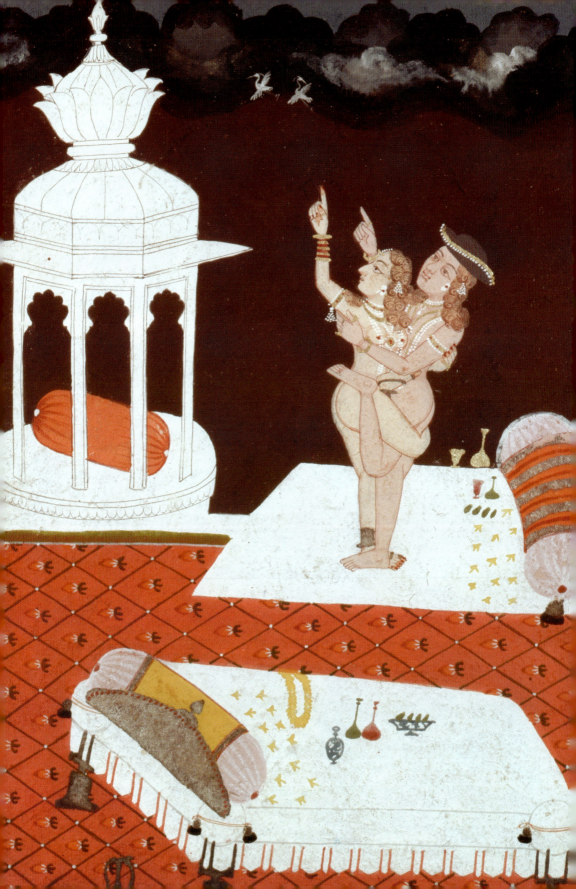

excitement of passion, and peculiarities of habit may sometime cause contrary results to appear, but these do not last long, and in the end the natural state is resumed

The wedge on the bosom, the scissors on the head, the piercing instrument on the cheeks, and the pinchers on the breasts and sides may also be taken into consideration with the other four modes of striking, and thus give eight ways altogether. But these four ways of striking with instruments are peculiar to the people of the southern countries, and the marks caused by them are seen on the breasts of their women. They are local peculiarities, but Vatsyayana is of the opinion that the practice of them is painful, barbarous, and base, and quite unworthy of imitation.

In the same way anything that is a local peculiarity should not always be adopted elsewhere, and even in the place where the practice is prevalent, excess of it should always be avoided. Instances of the dangerous use of them may be given as follows. The King of the Panchalas killed the courtesan Madhavasema by means of the wedge during congress. King Shatakarrni of the Kuntalas deprived his great Queen Malayavati of her life by a pair of scissors, and Naradeva, whose hand was deformed, blinded a dancing girl by directing a piercing instrument in a wrong way.

Facing page: Desire and eroticism are two sides of the same coin.

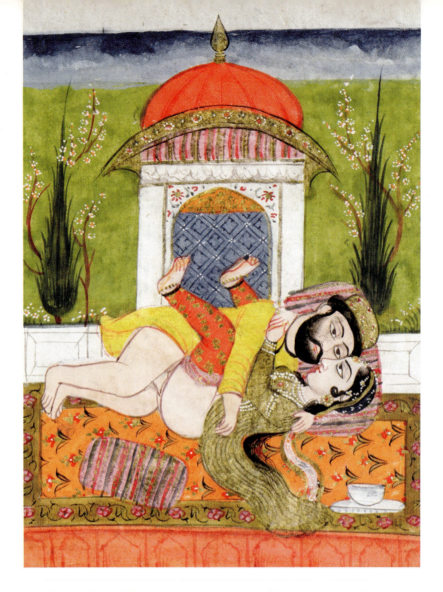

About these things there cannot be either enumeration or any definite rule. Congress having once commenced, passion alone gives birth to all the acts of the parties.

Such passionate actions and amorous gesticulations or movements which arise on the spur of the moment, and during sexual intercourse, cannot be defined, and are as irregular as dreams. A horse having once attained the fifth

Desire begins in the mind that contemplates physical intimacy with the loved one.

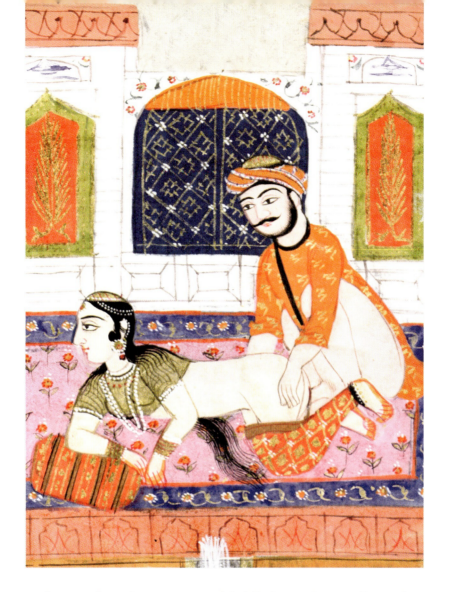

degree of motion goes on with blind speed, regardless of pits, ditches, and posts in his way; and in the same manner a loving pair become blind with passion in the heat of congress, and go on with great impetuosity paying not the least regard to excess. For this reason one who is well acquainted with the science of love, and knowing his own strength as also the tenderness, impetuosity, and strength of the young woman, should act accordingly. The various

At the height of passion, the notion of excesses becomes blurred.

modes of enjoyment are not for all times or for all persons, but they should only be used at the proper time, and in the proper countries and places.

⚜ ESSAYING NEW ROLES ⚜

When a woman sees that her lover is fatigued by constant congress, without having his desire satisfied, she should, with his permission, lay him down upon his back, and give him assistance by acting his part. She may also do this to satisfy the curiosity of her lover, or her own desire of novelty.

There are two ways of doing this, the first is when during congress she turns round, and gets on the top of her lover, in such a manner as to continue the congress, without obstructing the pleasure of it; and the other is when she acts the man's part from the beginning. At such a time, with flowers in her hair hanging loose, and her smiles broken by hard breathings, she should press upon her lover's bosom with her own breasts, and lowering her head frequently should do in return the same actions which he used to do before, returning his blows and chaffing him, should say, 'I was laid down by you, and fatigued with hard congress, I shall now therefore lay you down in return.'

Facing page: Vatsyayana strongly advocates the reversal of roles in the act of love.

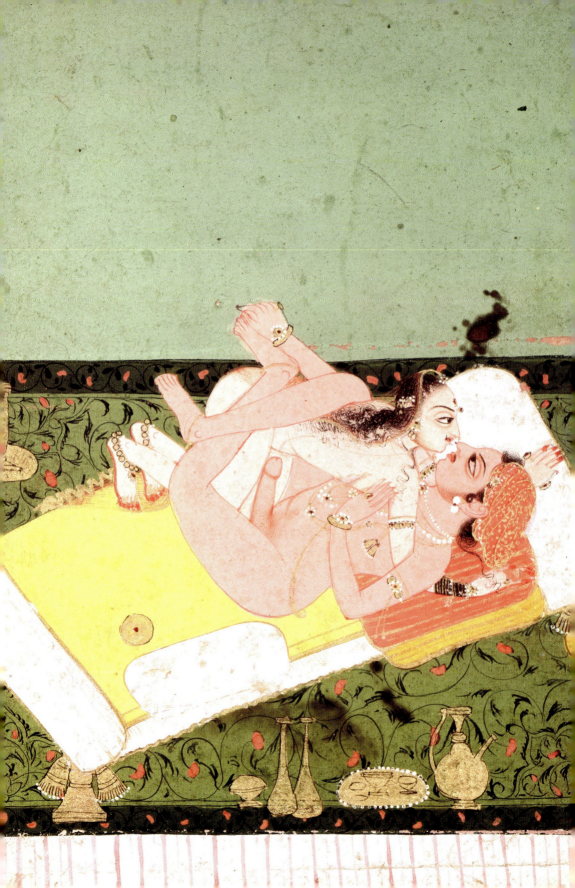

She should then again manifest her own bashfulness, her fatigue, and her desire of stopping the congress. In this way she should do the work of a man, which we shall presently relate.

What a man does for giving pleasure to a woman is called 'the work of a man', and is as follows:

While the woman is lying on his bed, and is as it were distracted by his conversation, he should loosen the knot of her undergarments, and when she begins to dispute with him, he should overwhelm her with kisses. Then when his *lingam* is erect he should touch her with his hands in various places, and gently manipulate various parts of the body. If the woman is bashful, and if it is the first time that they have come together, the man should place his hands between her thighs, which she would probably keep close together, and if she is a very young girl, he should first get his hands upon her breasts, which she would probably cover with her own hands, and under her armpits and on her neck. If, however, she is a seasoned woman, he should do whatever is fitting for the occasion. After this he should take hold of her hair, and hold her chin in his fingers for the purpose of kissing her. On this, if she is a young girl, she will become bashful and close her eyes. Anyhow he should gather from the action of the woman what things would be pleasing to her during congress.

When a woman is exhausted, she should place her forehead on that of her lover, and should thus take rest without disturbing the union of the organs, and when the woman has rested herself, the man should turn around and begin congress again.

Some verses on the subject are as under:

Though a woman is reserved, and keeps her feelings concealed, yet when she gets on top of a man, she then shows all her love and desire. A man should gather from the actions of the woman of what disposition she is, and in what way she likes to be enjoyed. A woman during her monthly courses, a woman who has been lately confined, and a fat woman should not be made to act the part of a man.

Here Suvarnanabha tells us that while a man is doing to the woman what he likes best during congress, he should always make a point of pressing those parts of her body on which she turns her eyes. The signs of the enjoyment and satisfaction of the woman are as follows:

Her body relaxes, she closes her eyes, she puts aside all bashfulness, and shows increased willingness to unite the

Following pages 164-165: A man who proceeds according to the inclinations of his woman would forever enjoy a passionate relationship.

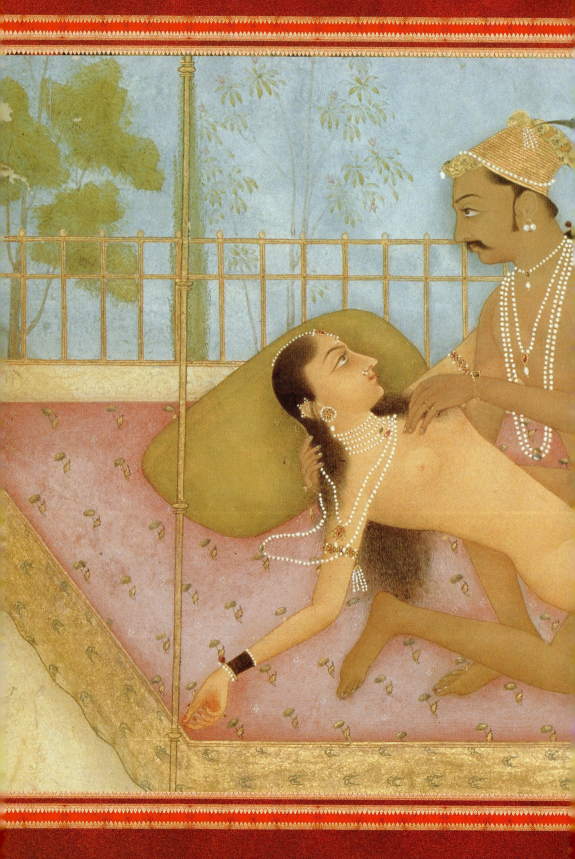

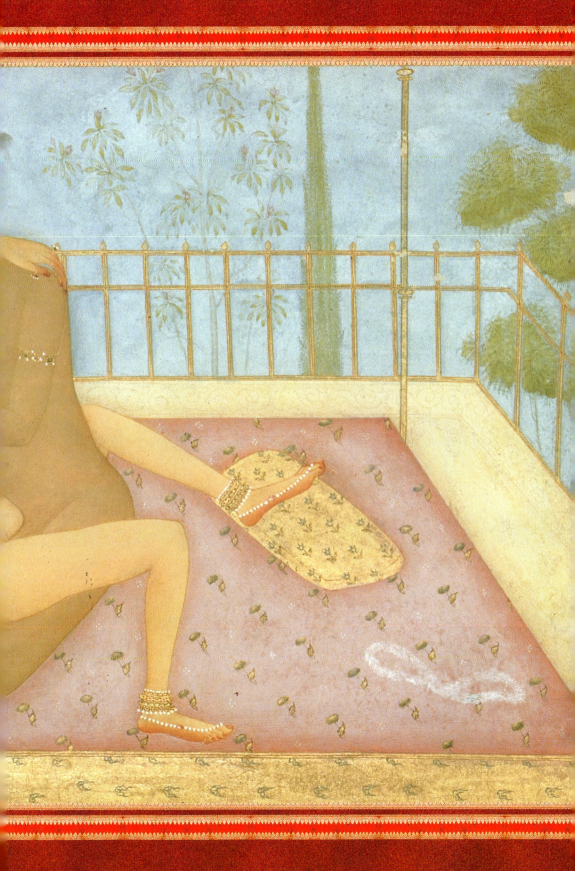

two organs as closely together as possible. On the other hand, the signs of her want of enjoyment and of failing to be satisfied are as follows: she shakes her hands, she does not let the man get up, feels dejected, bites the man, kicks him, and continues to go on moving after the man has finished. In such cases the man should rub the *yoni* of the woman with his hand and fingers (as the elephant rubs anything with his trunk) before engaging in congress, until it is softened, and after that is done he should proceed to put his *lingam* into her.

While Vatsyayana does defines roles for the man and the woman during the act of love, it is to be understood that these are not rules cast in stone. They are to be perceived, less as prescriptions and more as a list of suggestions that partners could follow in order to put each other at ease. The acts, then, to be done by the man are:

♣ MOVING FORWARD ♣

When the organs are brought together properly and directly it is called 'moving the organ forward'.

♣ FRICTION OR CHURNING ♣

When the *lingam* is held with the hand, and turned all round in the *yoni*, it is called 'churning'.

✤ PIERCING ✤

When the *yoni* is lowered and the upper part of it is struck with the *lingam*, it is called 'piercing'.

✤ RUBBING ✤

When the same thing is done on the lower part of the *yoni* it is called 'rubbing'.

✤ PRESSING ✤

When the *yoni* is pressed by the *lingam* for a long time, it is called 'pressing'.

✤ GIVING A BLOW ✤

When the *lingam* is removed to some distance from the *yoni* and then forcibly strikes it, it is called 'giving a blow'.

✤ THE BLOW OF A BOAR ✤

When only one part of the *yoni* is rubbed with the *lingam* it is called the 'blow of boar'.

✤ THE BLOW OF A BULL ✤

When both sides of the *yoni* are rubbed in this way, it is called the 'blow of a bull'.

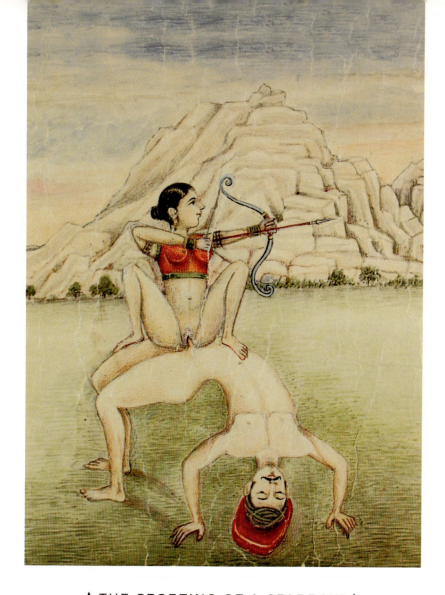

✤ THE SPORTING OF A SPARROW ✤

When the *lingam* is in the *yoni*, and is moved up and down frequently, and without being taken out, it is called the 'sporting of a sparrow'. This takes place at the end of congress.

When the roles are reversed and the woman acts the part of a

Mastering postures requires patience, passion and understanding between partners.

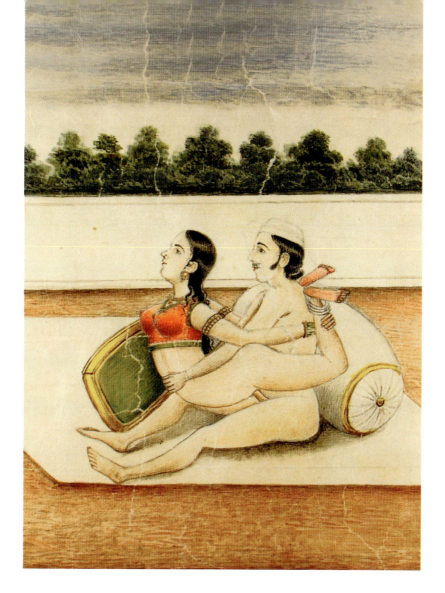

man, she has the following things to do in addition to the nine previously mentioned:

✣ THE PAIR OR TONGS ✣

When the woman holds the *lingam* in her *yoni*, draws it in, presses it, and keeps it in her for a long time, it is called the 'pair of tongs'.

When the wheels are set in motion, the chariots of desire roll on.

✤ THE TOP ✤

When, while engaged in congress, she turns round like a wheel, it is called the 'top'. This is learnt by practice only.

✤ THE SWING ✤

When, on such an occasion, the man lifts up the middle part of his body and the woman turns round her middle part it is called the 'swing'.

> When the woman is tired, she should place her forehead on that of her lover, and should thus take rest without disturbing the union of the organs, and when the woman has rested herself the man should turn round and begin the congress again.

✤ THE *AUPARISHTAKA* OR MOUTH CONGRESS ✤

> There are two kinds of eunuchs, those that are disguised as males, and those that are disguised as females. Eunuchs disguised as females imitate their dress, speech, gesture tenderness, timidity, simplicity, softness and bashfulness. The acts that are done on the *jaghana* or middle parts of women are done in the mouths of these eunuchs, and this

Facing page: A woman on top reveals to her man a sensual and passionate side to her that usually remains veiled.

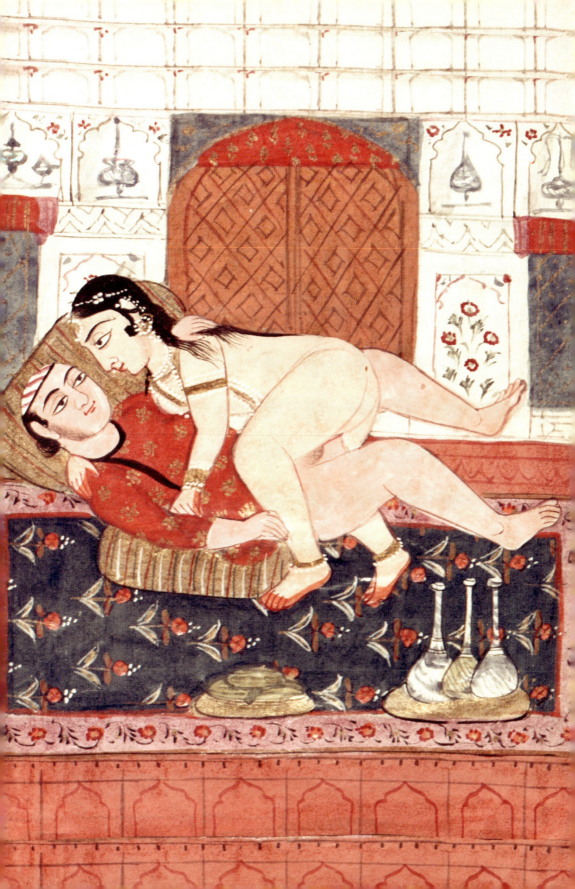

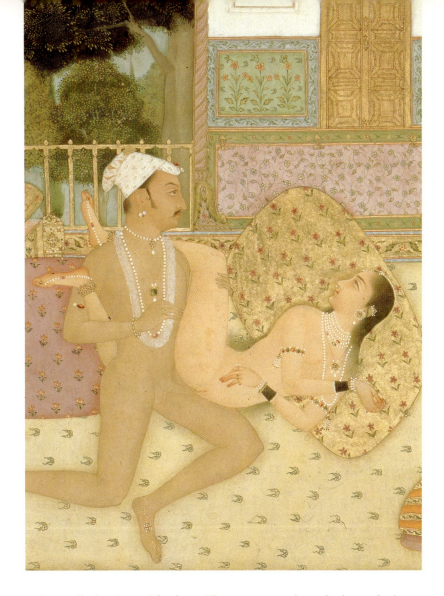

is called *Auparishtaka*. These eunuchs derive their imaginative pleasure, and their livelihood from this kind of congress, and they lead the life of courtesans. So much concerning eunuchs disguised as females.

Eunuchs disguised as males keep their desires secret, and when they wish to anything they lead the life of shampooers. Under the pretence of shampooing, a eunuch

---

In love there are no inhibitions, boundaries or limits.

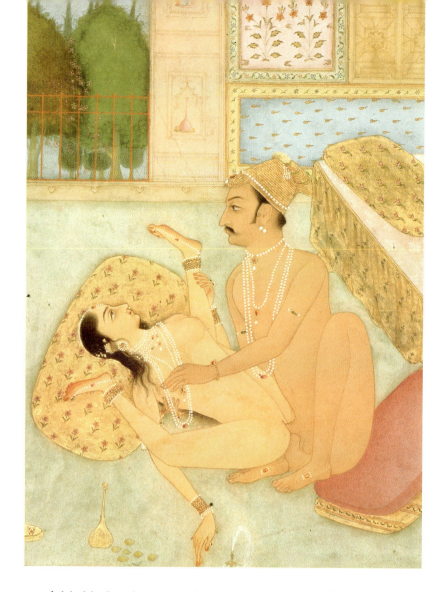

of this kind embraces and draws towards himself the thighs of the man whom he is shampooing, and after this he touches the joints of his thighs and his *jaghana* or central portion of his body. Then, if he finds the *lingam* of the man erect, he presses it with his hands, and chaffs him for getting into that state. If after this, and after knowing his intention, the man does not tell the eunuch to proceed, then the latter does it of his own accord and begins the congress. If,

A woman progressively reveals to her lover the manner in which she likes to be pleasured.

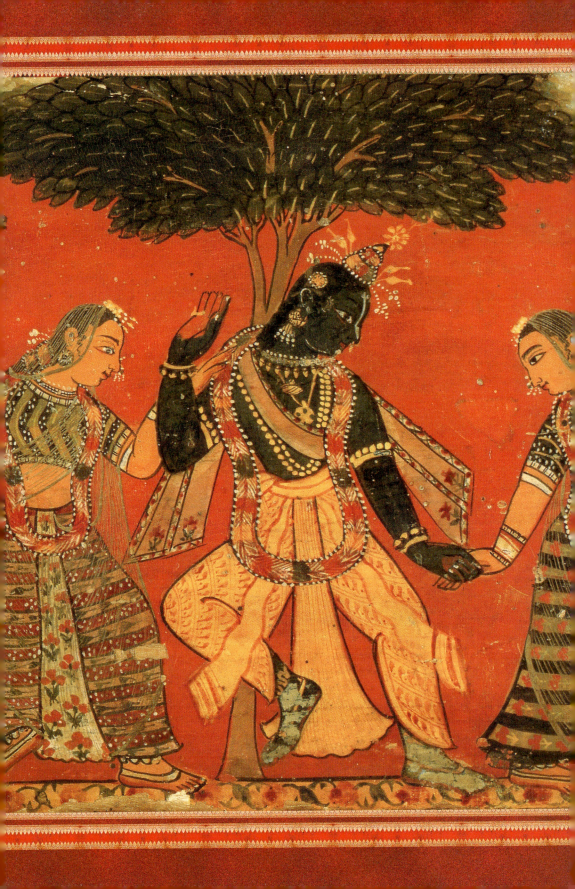

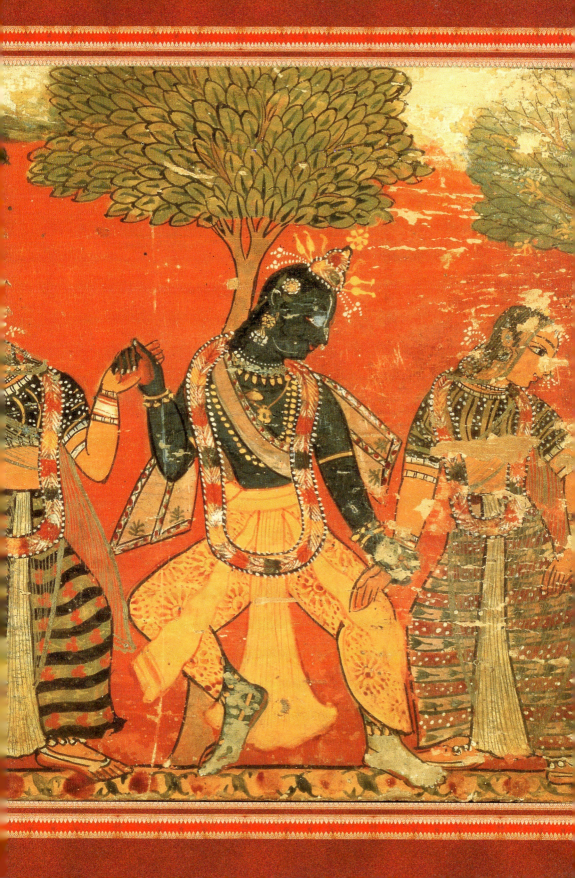

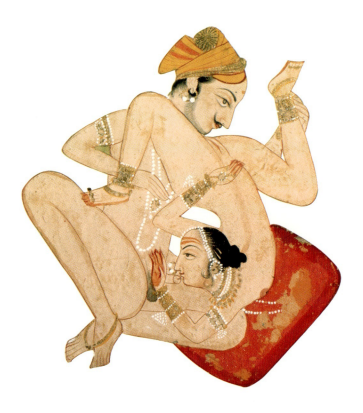

however, he is ordered by the man to do it, then he disputes with him, and only consents at last with difficulty.

The following eight things are then done by the eunuch one after the other:

At the end of each of these, the eunuch expresses his wish to stop, but when one of them is finished, the man desires

---

One of the greatest sources of sexual satisfaction is being pleasured by the partner's mouth. Preceding pages 174-175: Those who enjoy a healthy and passionate sexual relationship with their partners know how to spread love.

him to do another, and after that is done, then the one that follows it and so on.

♣ THE NOMINAL CONGRESS ♣

When, holding the man's *lingam* with his hand, and placing it between his lips, the eunuch moves about his mouth, it is called 'the nominal congress'.

♣ BITING THE SIDES ♣

When, covering the end of the *lingam* with his fingers collected together like the bud of a plant or flower, the eunuch presses the sides of it with his lips, using his teeth also, it is called 'biting the sides'.

♣ PRESSING OUTSIDE ♣

When, being desired to proceed, the eunuch presses the end of the *lingam* with his lips closed together, and kisses it as if he were drawing it out, it is called the 'outside pressing'.

♣ PRESSING INSIDE ♣

When, being asked to go on, he puts the *lingam* further into his mouth, and presses it with his lips and then takes it out, it is called the 'inside pressing'.

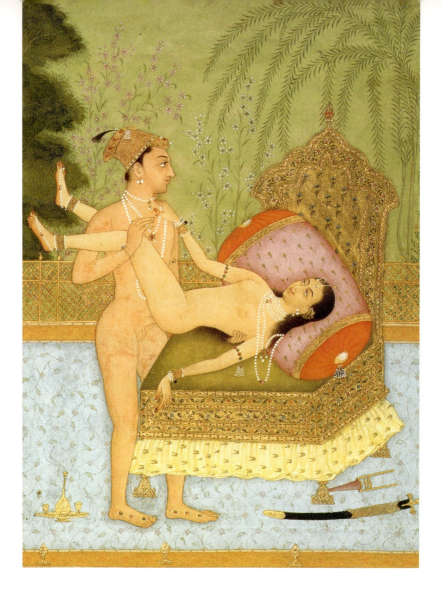

✤ KISSING ✤

When, holding the *lingam* in his hand, the eunuch kisses it as if he were kissing the lower lip, it is called 'kissing'.

✤ RUBBING ✤

When, after kissing it, he touches it with his tongue

A woman alternates between agony and ecstasy during the act of love.

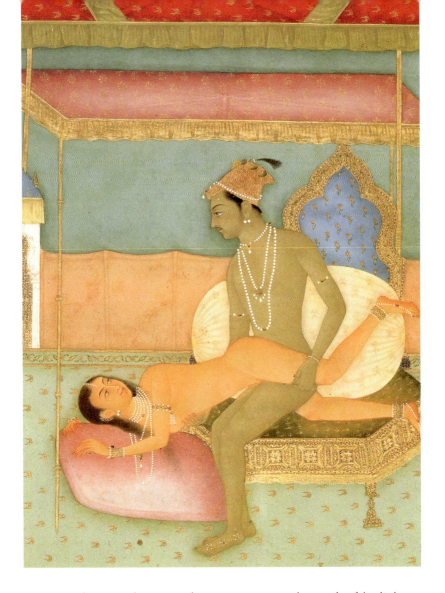

everywhere and passes the tongue over the end of it, it is called rubbing.

✦ SUCKING A MANGO FRUIT ✦

When, in the same way, he puts the half of it into his mouth and forcibly kisses and sucks it, this is called 'sucking a mango fruit'.

Mutual desire and passion constitute an important step to eliminating power games between a man and a woman.

✤ SWALLOWING UP ✤

And lastly, when, with the consent of the man, the eunuch puts the whole *lingam* into his mouth, and presses it to the very end, as if he were going to swallow it up, it is called 'swallowing it up'.

Striking, scratching, and other things may also be done during this kind of congress.

The *auparishtaka* is practised also by unchaste and wanton women, female attendants and serving maids, *i.e.*, those who are not married to anybody, but who live by shampooing.

The *acharyas* (ancient and venerable authors) are of opinion that this *auparishtaka* is the work of a dog and not of a man, because it is a low practice, and opposed to the orders of the Holy Writ, and because the man himself suffers by bringing his *lingam* into contact with the mouths of eunuchs and women.

But Vatsyayana tells us that:

The orders of the Holy Writ do not affect those who resort to courtesans, and the law prohibits the practice of the

Facing page: Men look for love; woman too look for love.

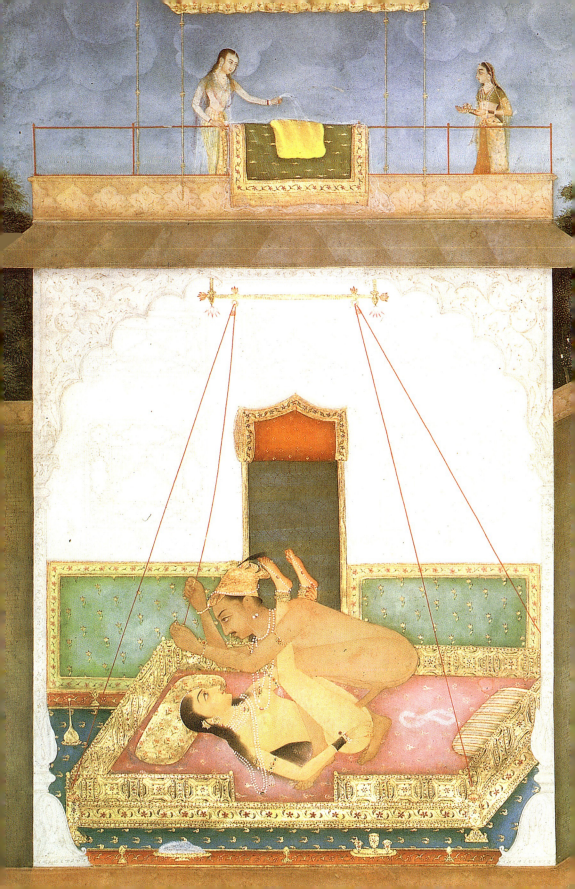

auparishtaka with married women only. As regards the injury to the male, that can be easily remedied.

The people of Eastern India do not resort to women who practise the *auparishtaka*.

The people of Ahichhatra resort to such women, but do nothing with them so far as the mouth is concerned.

The people of Saketa do with these women every kind of mouth congress, while the people of Nagara do not practise this, but do every other thing.

The people of the Shurasena country, on the southern bank of the Jumna, do everything without any hesitation, for they say that women no one can be certain about their character, their purity, their conduct, their practices, their confidences, or their speech. They are not however on this account to be abandoned, because religious law, on the authority of which they are reckoned pure, lays down that the udder of a cow is clean at the time of milking, though the mouth of a cow, and also the mouth

This and facing page: A woman in love contemplates fresh pleasures as she waits for her lover.

of her calf, are considered unclean by the Hindus. Again, a dog is clean when he seizes a deer in hunting, though food touched by a dog is otherwise considered very unclean. A bird is clean when it causes a fruit to fall from a tree by pecking at it, though things eaten by crows and other birds are considered unclean. And the mouth of a woman is clean for kissing and such like things at the time of sexual intercourse. Vatsyayana moreover thinks that in all these things connected with love, everybody should act according to the custom of his country, and his own inclination.

The male servants of some men carry on the mouth congress with their masters. Some citizens, who know each other well, among themselves, also practice it. Some women of the harem, when they are amorous, do the acts of the mouth on the *yoni*s of one another, and some men do the same thing with women. The way of doing this (kissing the

Following pages 184-185: A well-decorated and well-perfumed setting provides a perfect backdrop to lovemaking.

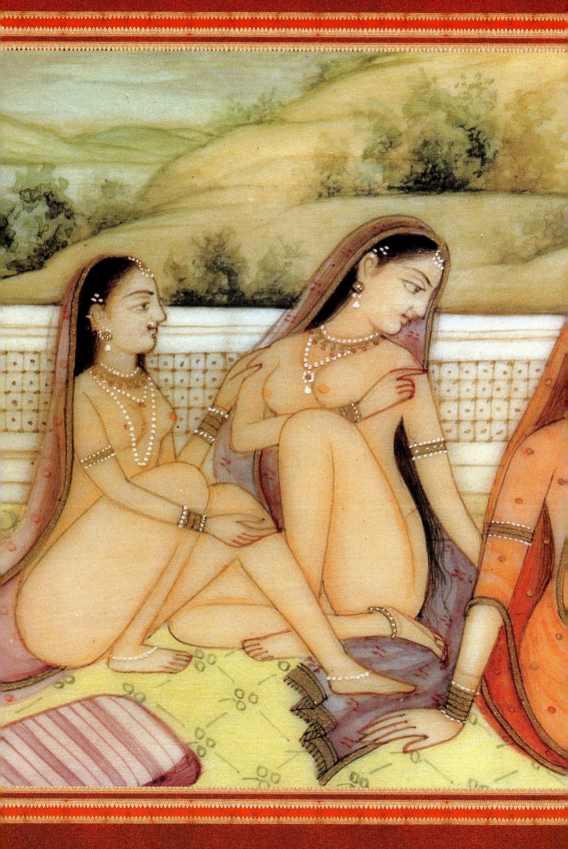

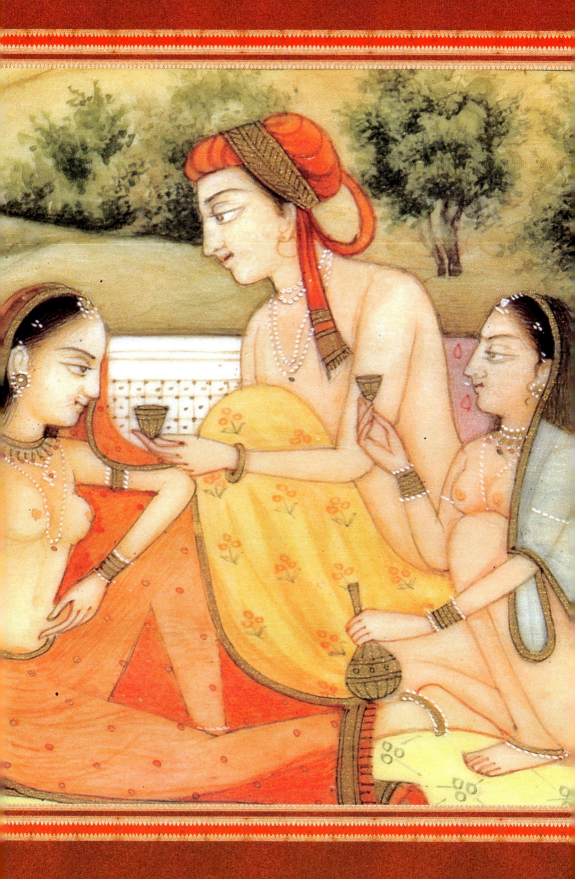

yoni) should be known from kissing the mouth. When a man and woman lie down in an inverted order, with the head of the one towards the feet of the other and carry on this congress, it is called the 'congress of a crow'.

For the sake of such things, courtesans abandon men possessed of good qualities, liberal and clever, and become attached to low persons, such as slaves and elephant drivers. The *auparishtaka*, or mouth congress, should never be done by a learned Brahman, by a minister that carries on the business of a state, or by a man of good reputation, because though the practice is allowed by the Shastras, there is no reason why it should be carried on, and need only be practised in particular cases. As for instance the taste, and the strength, and the digestive qualities of the flesh of dogs are mentioned in works on medicine, but it does not therefore follow that it should be eaten by the wise. In the same way there are some men, some places and some times, with respect to which these practices can be made use of. A man should therefore pay regard to the place, to the time, and to the practice, which is to be carried out, as also as to whether it is agreeable to his nature and to himself, and then he may or may not practise these things according to circumstances. But after all, these things being done secretly, and the mind of the man being fickle, how can it be known what any person will do at any particular time and for any particular purpose.'

♣ BEYOND LOVE AND HATE ♣

In the pleasure-room, decorated with flowers, and fragrant with perfumes, attended by his friends and servants, the man should receive the woman, who will come bathed and dressed, and will invite her to take refreshment and to drink freely. He should then seat her on his left side, and holding her hair, and touching also the end and knot of her garment, he should gently embrace her with his right arm. They should then carry on an amusing conversation on various subjects, and may also talk suggestively of things, which would be considered as coarse, or not to be mentioned generally in society. They may then sing, either with or without gesticulations, and play on musical instruments, talk about the arts, and persuade each other to drink. At last when the woman is overcome with love and desire, the citizen should dismiss the people that may be with him, giving them flowers, ointments, and betel leaves, and then when the two are left alone, they should proceed as has been already described in the previous chapters.

Such is the beginning of sexual union. At the end of the congress, the lovers, with modesty, and not looking at each other, should go separately to the washing-room. After this, sitting in their own places, they should eat some betel leaves, and the citizen should apply with his own hand to the body of the woman some pure sandalwood ointment, or ointment of some other kind. He should then embrace her with his left arm, and with agreeable words should cause her to drink from a cup held in his own hand, or he may give her water to drink. They can then eat sweetmeats or anything else, according to their liking, and may drink fresh juice, soup, gruel, extracts of meat, sherbet, the juice of mango fruits, the extract of the juice of the citron tree mixed with sugar, or anything that may be liked in different countries, and known to be sweet, soft, and pure. The lovers may also sit on the terrace of the palace or house, and enjoy the moonlight, and carry on an agreeable conversation. At this time too, while the woman lies in his lap, with her face towards the moon, the citizen should show her the different planets, the morning star, the polar star, and the seven Rishis, or Great Bear.'

This is the end of sexual union.

Congress is of the following kinds:

♣ LOVING CONGRESS ♣

When a man and a woman, who have been in love with each other for some time, come together with great difficulty, or when one of the two returns from a journey,

---

Facing page: Love is a playful and harmless game whose prime aim is bliss.

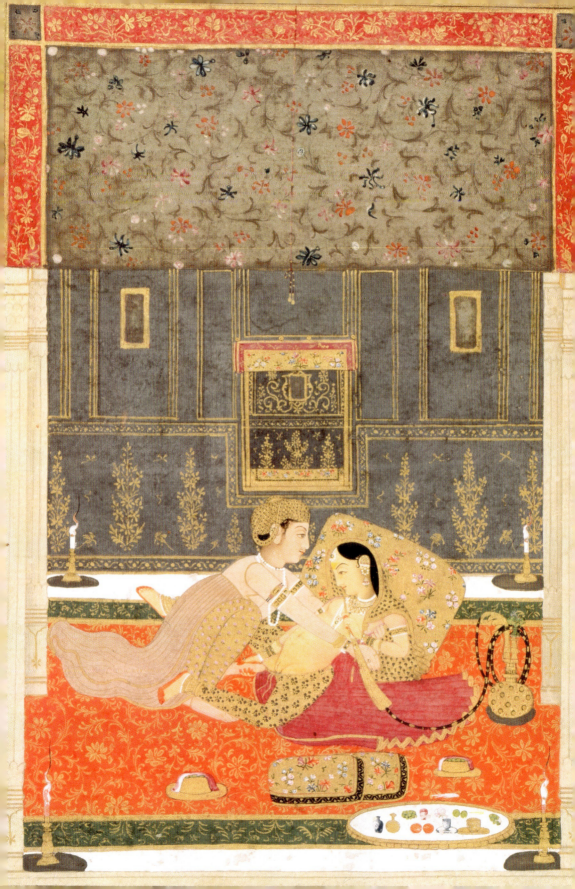

or is reconciled after having been separated on account of a quarrel, then congress is called the 'loving congress'. It is carried on according to the liking of the lovers, as long as they choose.

♣ CONGRESS OF SUBSEQUENT LOVE ♣

When two persons come together, while their love for each other is still in its infancy, their congress is called the 'congress of subsequent love'.

♣ CONGRESS OF ARTIFICIAL LOVE ♣

When a man carries on the congress by exciting himself by means of the sixty-four ways, such as kissing, etc., or when a man and a woman come together, though in reality they are both attached to different persons, their congress is then called 'congress of artificial love'. At this time all the ways and means mentioned in the Kama Shastra should be used.

♣ CONGRESS OF TRANSFERRED LOVE ♣

When a man, from the beginning to the end of the congress, though having connection with the woman, thinks all the time that he is enjoying another one whom he loves, it is called the 'congress of transferred love'.

♣ CONGRESS LIKE THAT OF EUNUCHS ♣

Congress between a man and a female water carrier, or a female servant of a caste lower than his own, lasting only until the desire is satisfied, is called 'congress like that of eunuchs'. Here external touches, kisses, and manipulations are not to be employed.

♣ DECEITFUL CONGRESS ♣

The congress between a courtesan and a rustic, and that between citizens and the women of villages, and bordering countries, is called 'deceitful congress'.

♣ CONGRESS OF SPONTANEOUS LOVE ♣

The congress that takes place between two persons who are attached to one another, and which is done according to their own liking is called 'congress of spontaneous love'.

Thus ends the kinds of congress. We shall now speak of lover's quarrels.

A woman who is very much in love with a man cannot bear to hear the name of her rival mentioned, or to have any conversation regarding her, or to be addressed by her name through mistake. If such takes place, a great quarrel arises, and the woman cries, becomes angry, tosses her hair about, strikes her lover, falls from her bed or seat, casting aside her garlands and ornaments, throws herself down on the ground.

At this time, the lover should attempt to reconcile her with conciliatory words, and should take her up carefully and place her on her bed. But she, not replying to his questions, and with increased anger, should bend down his head by pulling his hair, and having kicked him once, twice or thrice on his arms, head, bosom or back, should then proceed to the door of the room. She should then sit angrily near the door and shed tears, but should not go out, because she would be found

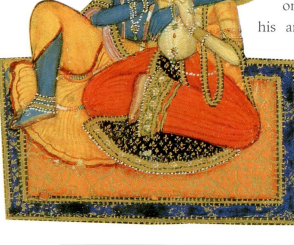

In love, there are no permanent disputes.

fault with for going away. After a time, when she thinks that the conciliatory words and actions of her lover have reached their utmost, she should then embrace him, talking to him with harsh and reproachful words, but at the same time showing a loving desire for congress.

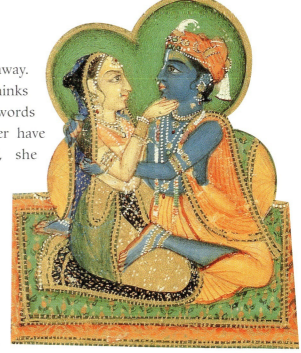

When a woman is in her own house, and has quarrelled with her lover, she should go to him and show how angry she is, and leave him. Afterwards the citizen having sent the Vita the Vidushaka or the Pithamurda to pacify her, she should accompany them back to the house, and spend the night with her lover.'

Thus ends the love quarrels.

Distance and discord are but renewers of love.

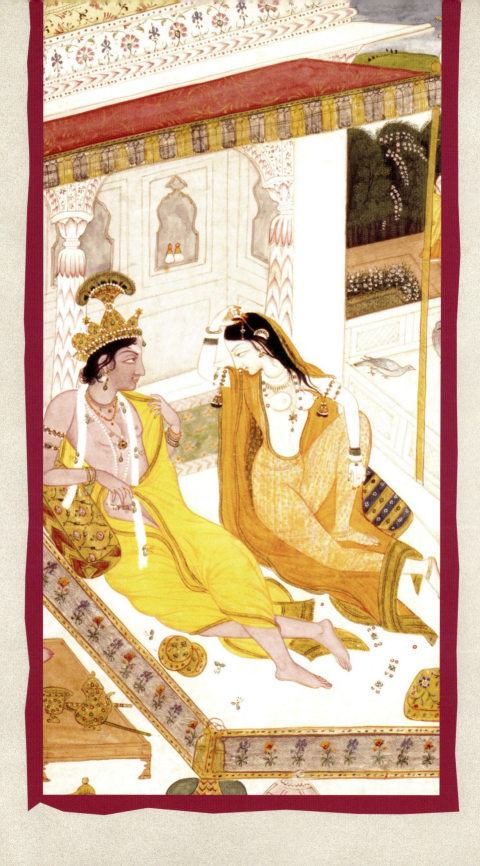

Conclusion: Towards Eternal Bliss

What is it that makes us turn the pages of a book compiled some two thousand years ago by a celibate ascetic? The essence lies perhaps in its understanding and presentation of a vast gamut of human relationships, and above all in the simplicity with which it teaches the reader, almost step by step, how to conduct oneself in a multi-layered and complex world.

Says Vatsyayana of the *Kama Sutra*: 'Although some learned men object,' yet he insists that women should read his work. He was writing for lovers, not just married people (like Kalyan Malla when he wrote the *Ananga Ranga*). It follows that the *Kama Sutra* is refreshingly open-minded and liberal in outlook. Perhaps this explains the book's enduring charm better than any other aspect.

As part of this debate amongst the scholars of yore, one group felt that there was no point in young women studying the art and practices laid out in the ancient texts. But Vatsayayna disagrees. He asserts that all women are instinctively aware of the practices of the *Kama Sutra*. And even though practice often leads to perfection, many, without understanding the science, become masters of the art.

Facing page: A woman is instinctively aware of the practices of love laid down in the Kama Sutra.

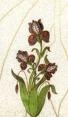

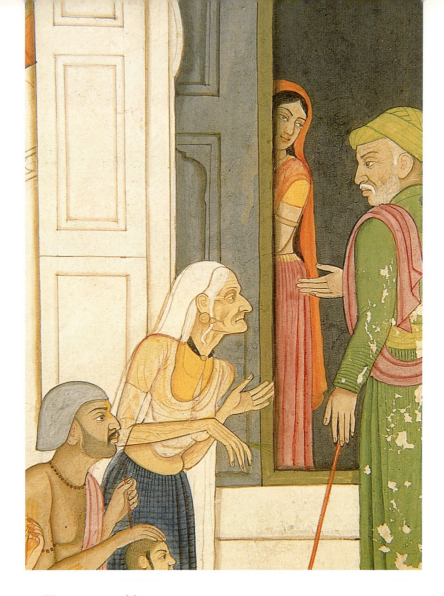

Vatsyayana adds:

Priests at times may not really understand the correct meaning of chants, but that does not stop them from worshipping the gods; horse-riders or elephant-mahouts train their charges without any formal training or knowledge of the science of training animals. In the

---

Elderly women are called upon to teach younger women about the arts.

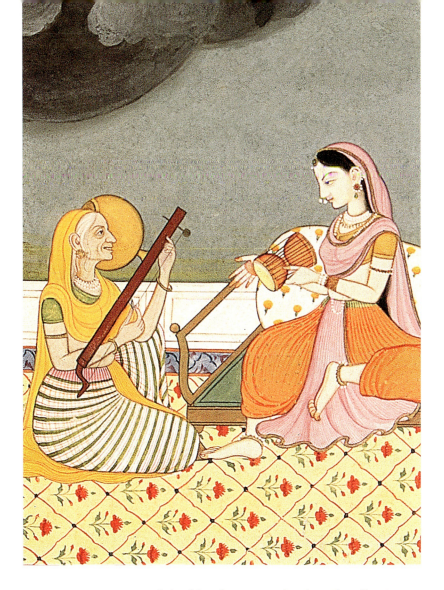

remotest corners of the kingdom, people obey the dictates of their king only because it is common practice. Similarly, highborn ladies and public women may be found to be well versed in ancient love treatises.

He strongly advises women to study the *Kama Sutra* or at least a part of it or learn it from a close confidante.

Proficiency in the arts ensures a mode of survival for a woman caught in difficult circumstances.

Study the sixty-four practices alone. The rest can be learnt from a teacher who must be from amongst the following: the daughter of a nurse brought up with you, already married; or another girl who can be trusted with almost anything; or an aunt, preferably your mother's sister; or an elderly maid; or a poor lady who had once lived with your family or your sister.

And that is not all, women are encouraged to learn to write in code or cipher or develop their own ways of writing.

It is important to learn new ways of speaking so that you can deftly change the beginning or end of words to suit your purpose. It's fun to be able to add unnecessary letters between every syllable of a word, or to be able to quibble. Learn to be especially skillful at language; it is a good mental exercise and can help you complete stanzas or verses that are incomplete; compose poems and with the use of a dictionary improve your vocabulary.

If you learn all there is to learn, you'll be given all the respect due to you by society and will be able to sit as an equal in an assembly of learned men. You will win the respect of the king and the praise of the wise; people will bend over backwards for your favours and you will be respected always.

> We are told that if a princess of royal lineage is well versed in these arts, she'll have no equal even if she were only one amongst her husband's thousand wives.
>
> Remember all these will be useful if for some reason you're separated from your husband and fall into bad times. You will have no cause for worry. These arts will help you even if you are stranded in a foreign land forlorn.

While the *Kama Sutra* stresses the need for young maidens and women to study it, it is not to be viewed simply as a codifying of the sixty-four postures that bring a woman and a man close to each other in the act of lovemaking. Of course these are described in detail but the purpose is not to titillate but to educate. For Vatsyayana goes far beyond the relationship between a man and woman that begins and ends in marriage. In the seven books of aphorisms—General Principles, Sexual Union, Courtship and Marriage, the Wife, Seducing the Wives of Others, Courtesans, and Erotic Love, he even explores heterosexuality.

Perhaps one of the reasons for the continuing appeal of this manual of love lies not just in its antiquity but on its essential modernity. Two thousand years ago, Vatsyayana wrote:

> Men look for love, women too look for love: women play the main role in the act of intercourse.

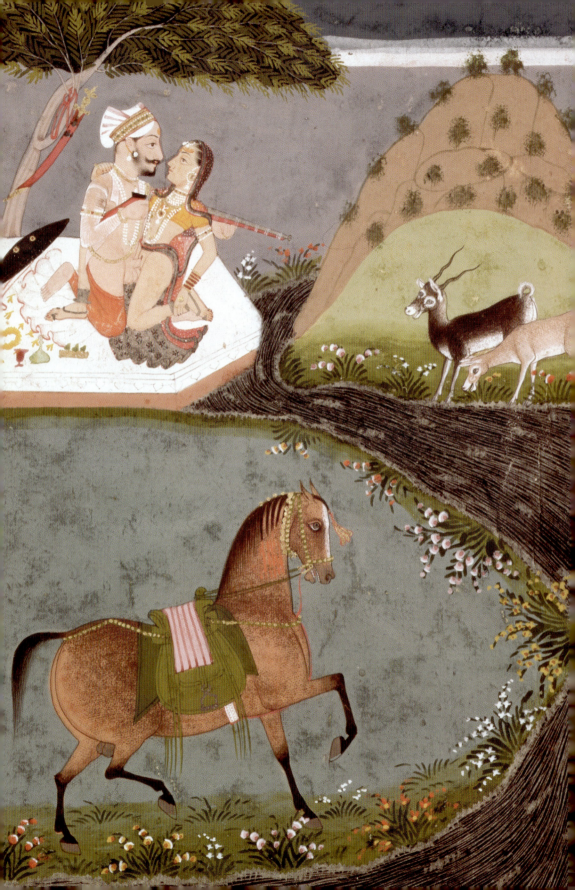

He sought to teach men to appreciate the sterling value of a liberated female. For she who is knowledgeable, is fulfilled. Without variety, the very springs of the life force would run dry and the river of life would get lost among the boulders of monotony. For physical intimacy was a necessary station to *ananda* or bliss. Should a couple fail to enjoy intimacy, sex would have no meaning. Thus each partner has to ensure that the embers of desire continue to glow, the incandescent fires of passion burn brightly after years of living with each other, and love flourishes.

In Vatsyayana's times, monogamy was the preferred norm and had as its bedrock, respect, love, faith and the right to find sexual satisfaction. But the sages of ancient India also knew that sometimes, sexual happiness could be the missing ingredient in an otherwise perfectly normal marriage. So they explored possibilities with multiple partners outside the institution of marriage.

If one were to delve into Indian mythology, one would stumble upon the *apsara* Menaka coming down to disrupt the *tapasya* of the hermit Vishwamitra or instances where the all-too-human gods nurse adulterous thoughts. Courtesans were respected for their expertise in the art of love. Casual relationships, contractual arrangements, relationships with housemaids, and houses of pleasure were all part of the social structure. The *Kama Sutra* gives human sexuality its rightful place in society and even examines

Facing page: Courtesans were respected for their mastery of the art of love.

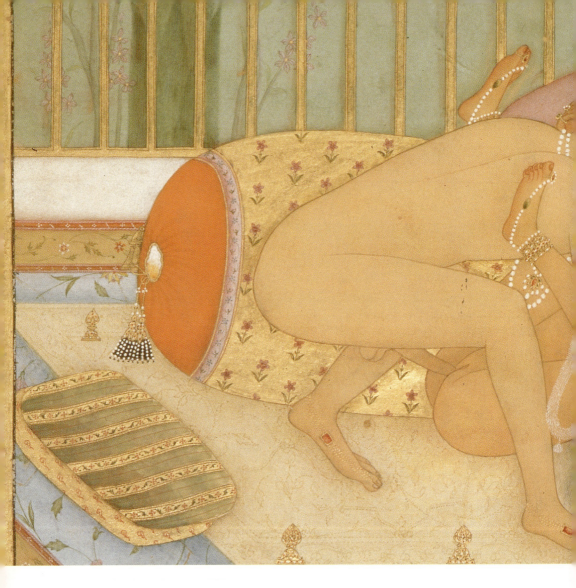

aspects of sexuality such as homosexuality, lesbianism, prostitututution, or persons of a 'third nature' and more.

Often, Vedic India is seen as an important milestone in the history of Indian womanhood. In this male-dominated society, in matters of sexual pleasure there was no separation between the needs of both men and women, for to take away that one prime ingredient from either would be to negate the fundamental purposes of nature. In a social milieu where equality was a matter

When women are treated as equals in love, the act of love itself becomes more than a fleeting episode.

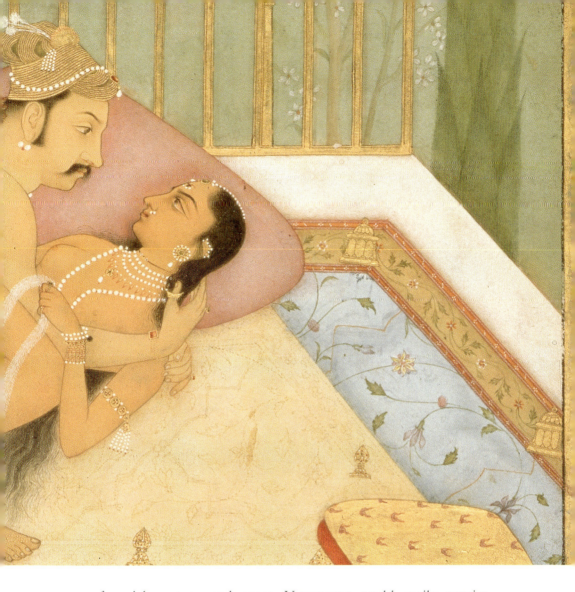

of social custom and grace, Vatsyayana could easily restrict himself to the fulcrum of pleasure and sexual fulfillment. He did not have to champion the rights of women or become an advocate of women's liberation—'When treated as equals, sexual intercourse becomes more than just a fleeting episode'.

The *Kama Sutra* teaches women not be content just being passive partners but to explore and demand sexual happiness and satisfaction.

In order to harmonize the relationship between men and women, it was men on whom the onus lay for concentrating on the gentle art of romance, courtship, seduction, foreplay and then sexual intercourse. So it taught them to be more considerate, more skillful in their relationship with not just their wives but with all women in general. Vatsyayana believed that there was an essential difference between the psychological mindset of the male and female in that, it was mostly men who took the lead while women assumed the passive role, for women were aroused slowly. Looking for a harmonious solution, he found that one should prefer a relationship with one's own kind or type. And this alchemy was a mixture of temperament, emotional make up, expectations or physical build.

Vatsyayana knew that if human relationships were to come to fruition, it was only the male who had to subdue his ego, and be more giving and selfless. Any courtship that had no consideration for the other partner was doomed before it began. Thus he laid stress upon skill, gentleness and foreplay. With this in mind, he guides the uninitiated into the realms of a woman's fantasy, which if properly applied could open the doors to mystical heights. For pleasure is a tender blossom that flowers with gentle care.

And lovemaking is not a one-way road. It's based on mutual pleasure. Vatsyayana puts it down thus:

> Every lover must reciprocate the beloved's gesture with equal intensity, kiss for kiss and embrace for embrace. If there is no reciprocity, the beloved will feel dejected and consider the lover as a stone-pillar. It will result in a highly

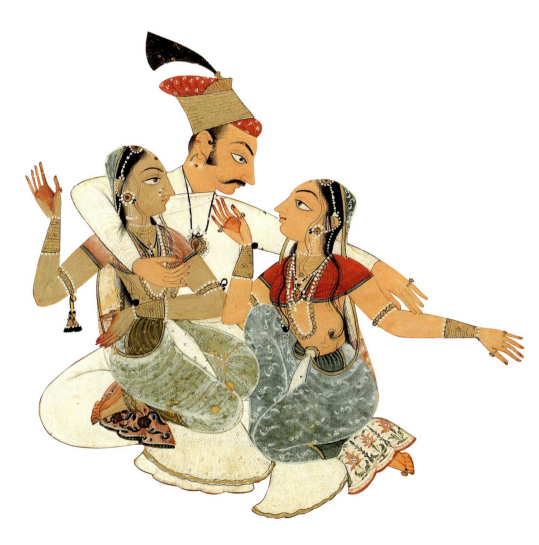

unsatisfactory union. To keep the passion alive and inflamed, reciprocity is absolutely essential.

In the great Game of Love, we are told:

Vatsyayana advises men to love and respect not only their wives but other women as well.

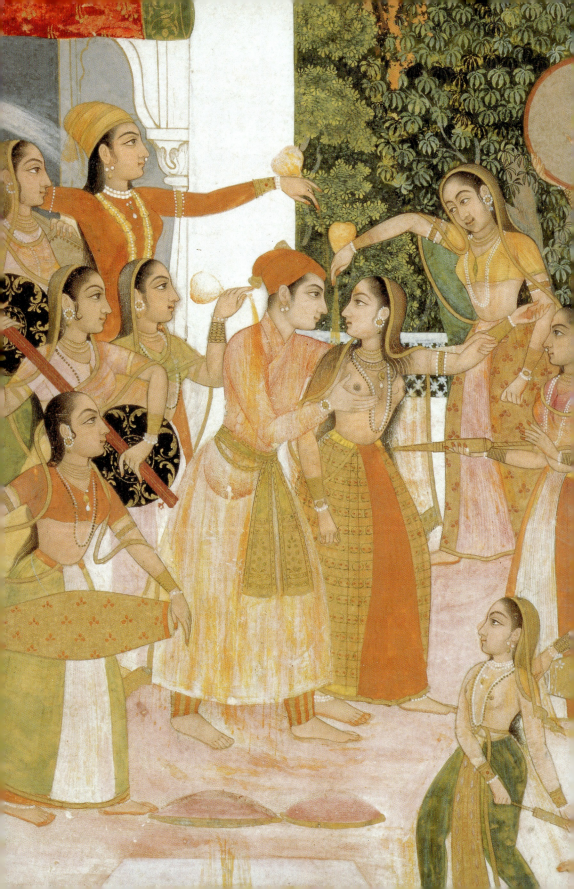

At all times, the man must carefully observe every action of the woman he loves, and so gauge her passion and preferences, and act accordingly, to give her the greatest pleasure.

The *Kama Sutra* opens the magical doors of sensuousness: to touch, to feel, to taste and to explore the eternal mysteries of the human body. To seek and to find the rapture in every single part of the human body—breasts, thighs, hips, eyes, lips, hair in an effort to be catapulted to 'the little death' or orgasm—the very acme of pleasure. Desire and eroticism are two sides of the same coin. They are an inseparable part of every individual's being. And once the floodgates are thrown open, pleasure remains the sole operating principle.

Facing page: Love is exploring the eternal mysteries of the human body and mind.

All rights reserved. No part of this publication
may be transmitted or reproduced in any form
or by any means without prior permission
from the publisher.

ISBN: 81-7436-440-4

© Roli & Janssen BV 2006
This edition published in 2006
in arrangement with
Roli & Janssen BV, The Netherlands
M-75 Greater Kailash II (Market)
New Delhi 110 048, India
Ph: ++91-11-29212782, 29210886
Fax: ++91-11-29217185
E-mail: roli@vsnl.com
Website: rolibooks.com

Design: Arati Subramanyam
Layout: Naresh Mondal
Production: Naresh Nigam

Printed and bound in Singapore

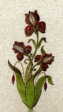